QUICK MEALS FOR A TACTICAL LIFE

SGT PEREZ
N. Alessandro Penington Books

COOKING W/SGT PEREZ

ISBN: 979-8-9898191-3-3 (Hardback)
ISBN: 979-8-9898191-4-0 (Paperback)

Front cover image by Perez MMG Publishing
Book design by Perez MMG Publishing

Printed in United States of America

First printing edition 2024.

Seerendip Publishing

Contents

Introduction

I'm Sergeant Perez, and I LOVE to cook and want to share some of my quick and easy recipes that I have been working on for some time now. In this book, you will find more than 30 easy-to-follow recipes that you can use anytime, anywhere to whip up some tasty grub. They're made with basic ingredients found anywhere in the world, so you won't need to lug around food or bottled water as you move through life—just throw in some fresh produce, stock up on canned goods, and pick up a bag of rice or dried pasta before your next mission!

If you're in the business of tactical operations, or just have a crazy busy life and you find yourself wondering how to make quick, easy meals that don't require hours of preparation, you've come to the right place! In my new cookbook "Quick and Easy Meals for a Tactical Life", you'll find 30+ time-saving recipes that are sure to satisfy your hunger and leave you enough time to plan your next operation... or watch your favorite sitcom! (Because let's face it, life isn't all about work.)

A lot of people these days are living very busy lives. That can mean that they don't always have time to cook themselves something good to eat. That doesn't mean they have to be stuck eating fast food all the time, though. There are some great ways to make healthy, tasty food quickly and easily. I, Sgt. Perez, will show you how with these quick tips! -So go clean out your fridge! You might find a few vegetables or fruits that need to be eaten up soon.

- **Plan:** Look at recipes online, write them down on index cards, or put together meal prep kits in advance so you're ready when hunger strikes.

- **Make it manageable:** Cook just one dish instead of making everything from scratch. Or just make a single pot of soup or chili if you want more than one course but less than four courses.

- **Cook together:** If there's someone else around who is hungry too, maybe the two of you can work together and tackle two dishes at once.

- **Use spices creatively:** They're not just meant to flavor food--spices are also healthy ingredients too! For those times when you don't have much time but want something hearty, delicious, and nutritious - these recipes are for you, Enjoy!

WHAT ARE QUICK MEALS?

In today's world, we're all living busy lives. We have jobs, families and other commitments that pull us in different directions. When time gets tight, it can be tough to find time to cook a healthy meal.

That's where quick meals come in handy! Quick meals are typically pre-packaged meals that you can find at your local grocery store or big box retailer like Costco. They're great because they require little preparation and offer balanced nutrition.

THE BENEFITS OF QUICK MEALS

- Flexible. Order when you want and eat it whenever you like – it's completely flexible as well as quick and easy!
- Easy. Ready meals are so easy!
- Pre-prepared!
- Nutritional Expertise!
- Satisfaction Guaranteed!
- Quality!
- Cost Effectiveness!

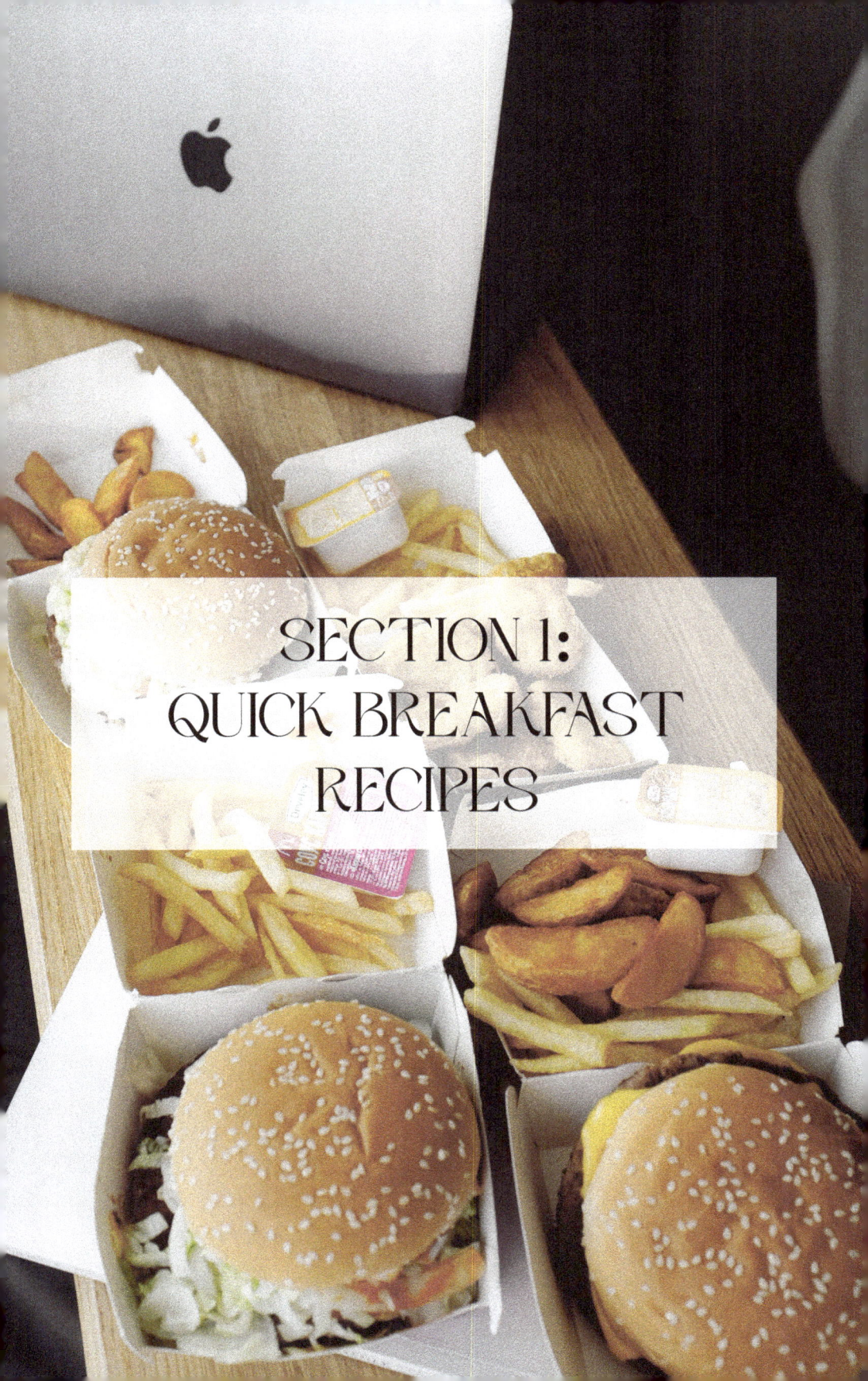

SECTION 1: QUICK BREAKFAST RECIPES

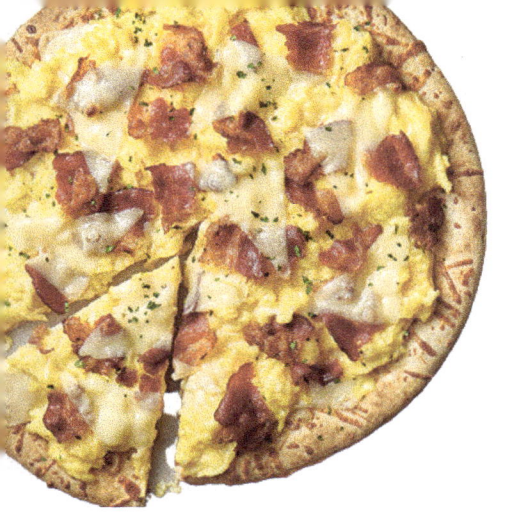

BACON & EGG PIZZA

This is one of my favorite quick meals. It's simple, fast, and delicious. I call this dish Bacon & Egg Pizza because it's basically pizza without sauce or cheese. It's the perfect recipe to make when you're in a hurry but still want something filling and tasty! Make your bacon crispy (I like to use a cast-iron skillet) and scramble eggs with salt, pepper, and fresh thyme leaves. Put a piece of whole wheat crust on an oven-safe plate and layer it with crispy bacon, scrambled eggs, and shredded mozzarella cheese. Bake for 10 minutes at 400 degrees Fahrenheit. Top with parsley. Sprinkle with lemon juice. Eat while it's hot.

Ingredients:

Eggs
- 8 large Land O Lakes Eggs
- 3 tablespoons milk
- 1 tablespoon Land O Lakes Butter

Pizza
- 1 (10-ounce) (11-inch) thin prepared pizza crust
- 6 (3/4-ounce) slices Land O Lakes Deli American, divided
- 4 slices bacon, crisply cooked, cut into 1-inch pieces

How to Make:

1. Heat oven to 450°F.
2. Whisk eggs and milk together in bowl.
3. Melt butter in 10-inch nonstick skillet; add egg mixture. Cook, lifting gently and stirring slightly to allow uncooked portions to flow underneath, 2-3 minutes or until set. Remove from heat; set aside.
4. Place pizza crust onto large baking sheet; top with 4 slices cheese, cooked eggs and bacon.
5. Cut remaining 2 slices cheese into quarters: separate pieces. Place cheese pieces over pizza. Bake 9-11 minutes or until cheese is melted.
6. Cut into 6 wedges. Serve hot.

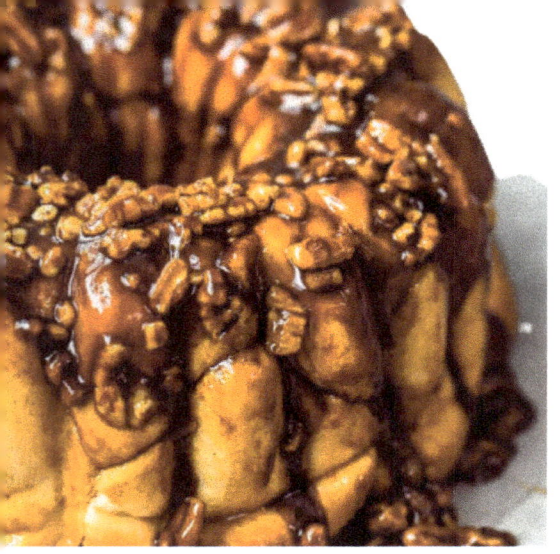

BUTTERSCOTCH MONKEY BREAD RECIPE

BUTTERSCOTCH MONKEY BREAD is a quick, easy dessert that takes about 45 minutes to make and serves 6-8 people. This recipe is a little different from most because I use butterscotch chips instead of traditional yellow cake mix.

Ingredients:

- 4 cups all-purpose flour
- 1 cup sugar
- 1 teaspoon salt
- 3 teaspoons baking powder
- 2 eggs
- ½ cup butter or margarine
- 1 teaspoon vanilla extract
- 2/3 cup milk
- 3.5 ounces Cook 'n Serve Butterscotch Pudding Mix 99 grams (1 box)
- ½ cup dark brown sugar 107 grams
- ¾ teaspoon ground cinnamon (or Penzey's pie spice)
- 1 cup chopped pecans 113 grams, divided (optional)
- 24 unbaked frozen dinner rolls 912 grams, Rhodes recommended

How to Make:

1. Generously spray a 10-inch Bundt pan with nonstick cooking spray.
2. Microwave the butter, butterscotch pudding mix, brown sugar, cinnamon, and salt on 50% power until butter has melted. Whisk together until incorporated.
3. ½ cup unsalted butter, 3.5 ounces Cook 'n Serve Butterscotch Pudding Mix, ½ cup dark brown sugar, ¾ teaspoon ground cinnamon, ¼ teaspoon kosher salt
4. Sprinkle ½ cup pecans into the pan.
5. 1 cup chopped pecans
6. Place half the frozen rolls evenly over the pecans leaving a little space (¼-inch) between rolls.
7. 24 unbaked frozen dinner rolls
8. Sprinkle the remaining ½ cup pecans and ½ of the butter/pudding mixture over the rolls.
9. Add the remaining frozen rolls on top of the butter/pudding mixture (cutting the rolls where needed).
10. Top evenly with the remaining butter/pudding mixture.
11. Spray one side of plastic wrap with nonstick spray and place it loosely (sprayed side down) over the rolls.
12. Leave the pan for 5-6 hours (on the countertop) or 8-10 hours (in the refrigerator).
13. When ready to bake, preheat oven to 350°F and bake 25-27 minutes, or until the internal temperature registers 200°F-205°F.
14. Transfer the pan to a cooling rack and cool 5 minutes.
15. Set a large plate (larger than the pan) over the rolls and invert the rolls onto the plate. Be very careful – the pan and the rolls are very hot, and the drippings can burn if not extremely careful.

Serve immediately.

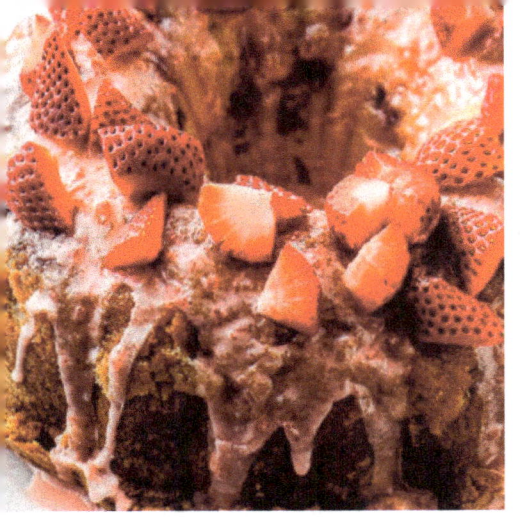

STRAWBERRY POUND CAKESTRAWBERRY POUND CAKE

This strawberry pound cake is a quick, easy, and delicious dessert that doesn't require much more than a few ingredients and about an hour in the oven. It is great served with whipped cream or vanilla ice cream!

Ingredients:

- 2 ½ cups of Strawberries
- 12oz Unsalted Butter
- 1 ¾ cup Sugar
- 5 Eggs
- 3 cups All-purpose Flour
- 1 tsp Baking Soda and Baking Powder
- 1 tsp Salt
- 1 Tbsp Lemon Zest
- 1 tsp Vanilla Extract
- 1 tsp Strawberry Extract (or you may replace it with Vanilla Extract)
- ¾ cup Sour Cream
- 2-3 tsp Red Food Coloring (Adds visual appeal)

How to Make:

1. Cream together the sugar and butter and add in the eggs.
2. Mix in the flour in batches and stir in the salt.
3. Mix in the half and half and flavorings.
4. Fold in the strawberries.
5. Bake and let cool.
6. Boil together the water and sugar and mix in the pureed strawberries.
7. Poke holes in the baked cake and pour over most of the strawberry syrup. Let the cake cool.
8. Make the strawberry glaze and drizzle over the cooled cake.

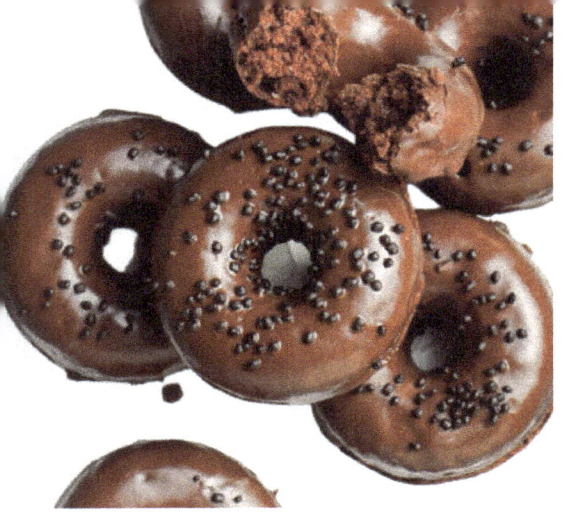

CHOCOLATE DOUGHNUT

Sometimes you need to get creative with what you have on hand. Chocolate donuts are an easy way to make a dessert or breakfast in a pinch. This recipe is based off my favorite boxed brownie mix and uses ingredients I always have on hand. The result is delicious! It's simple to make baked chocolate donuts at home with just 9 common ingredients! These chocolate donuts have a thick chocolate frosting and are soft and creamy.

Ingredients:

- ¾ cup All-purpose flour:
- 3 tbsp Cocoa powder:
- ½ cup Granulated sugar:
- 1 tsp baking powder:
- ¼ tsp Salt
- ¼ cup Vegetable oil:
- ½ cup Milk
- 3 tbsp Vanilla extract:
- 3 Eggs

How to Make:

1. Preheat the oven to 350ºF. Spray a donut pan with non-stick cooking spray then use a paper towel to evenly coat the entire donut well.

2. In a smaller bowl, combine the flour, cocoa powder, sugar, baking powder and salt, mix until combined. Set aside.

3. In a mixing bowl combine the milk, egg, vanilla extract and vegetable oil, use a whisk or spatula to beat. Gradually add the flour mixture, mixing by hand with a spatula just until combined.

4. Transfer the batter to a piping bag fit with a round piping tip and pipe the batter evenly into the donut wells. Use a small spatula to smooth the tops of the batter if the batter is uneven.

5. Bake for 10-13 minutes or until a toothpick inserted in the center of a donut comes out clean. Allow the donuts to cool for 10 minutes in the donut pan. Then turn the donut pan upside down and hit the pan against a counter a few times to release the donuts. Allow them to cool completely before dipping.

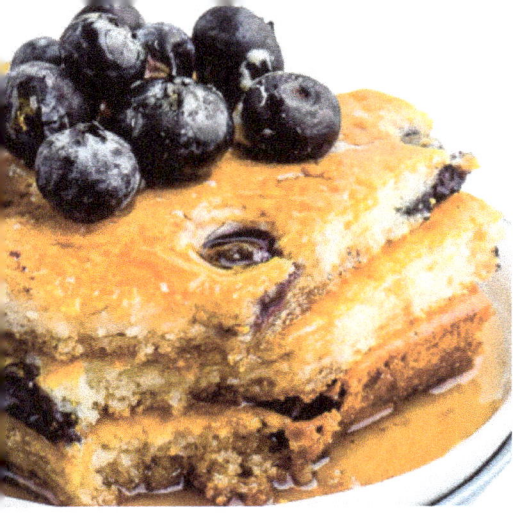

BLUEBERRY SHEET PAN PANCAKES

The tasty blueberry sheet pan pancake has made breakfast much easier and tastier. In under 30 minutes, it's ready and ideal for serving a crowd! Sheet pan recipes are simple to prepare and usually only require a few steps, allowing you to do something else besides stand at the stove cooking. It's time to start playing the sheet pan game with breakfast. Using a simple buttermilk pancake batter, this blueberry sheet pans recipe bakes in about 15 minutes. A delicious breakfast can be had by cutting the sheet pancakes into squares and serving them with butter and syrup.

Ingredients:

- 2 or 3 tablespoons neutral vegetable oil or melted butter, to grease sheet pan
- 1/2 cup unsalted butter, melted
- 1 1/4 cups milk
- 1 1/2 cups buttermilk
- 1 egg
- 1 teaspoon pure vanilla extract

- 3 cups all-purpose flour
- 1 tablespoon baking powder
- 1 teaspoon baking soda
- 3/4 teaspoon kosher salt
- 1/4 cup sugar
- 1 cup blueberries or add-ins of choice
- Maple syrup and softened butter, to serve

How to Make:

1. Preheat the oven to 450°F and grease a half-sheet pan with melted butter or neutral vegetable oil. Be sure the grease the sides, too.
2. Whisk together the milk, buttermilk, egg, and vanilla extract. Whisk a few tablespoons of the milk mixture into the melted butter to temper, and then pour the tempered butter into the liquid. Whisk to fully combine.
3. In a large mixing bowl, combine the flour, baking powder, baking soda, salt, and sugar. Add the liquid to the dry ingredients and use a spatula to stir, just until combined. It's ok if there are a few lumps.
4. Place the greased sheet pan in the oven and heat for a solid 5 minutes

while the pancake batter stands, and you pour yourself a fresh cup of coffee.

5. Taking care not to burn yourself, remove the hot pan from the oven and place it on a cooling rack or trivet. Pour the pancake batter into the sheet pan and spread evenly. Sprinkle the blueberries or any toppings of choice all over.
6. Bake for 13 to 15 minutes, until the pancake is baked through and the center springs back when lightly pressed, like a cake.
7. Change the oven setting to broil. Place the pancake under the broiler and brown the top. This will take around 1 or 2 minutes but check almost constantly; it will brown very fast.
8. Cut into squares and serve hot with butter and syrup.

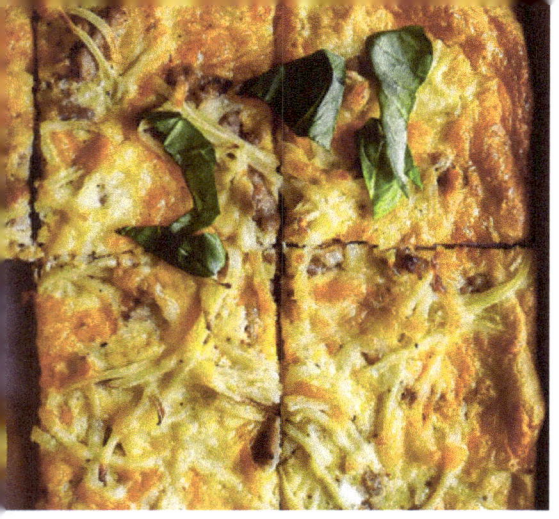

BREAKFAST PIZZA RECIPE (SHEET PAN)

One of the family's favorite morning dishes is breakfast pizza! This pizza is delicious and filling, from the crescent roll crust to the eggs and cheese within, and everything in between. Plus, since this pizza is prepared in a sheet pan, it is quite simple to make.

This pizza makes a delectable centerpiece for a brunch table during the holidays or for a weekend brunch. My love for breakfast pizza dates to my early years. I enjoy experimenting with new breakfast recipes every Christmas.

A popular simple breakfast recipe is sheet pan breakfast pizza! This pizza is filling and simple to create, from the crescent roll crust to the eggs and cheese within, and everything in between!

Ingredients:

- 1 pkg. Crescent Rolls
- 8 ounces Jimmy Dean Sausage – (regular, hot or maple) (you can use more or less to adjust to your taste preference)
- 1 cup Shredded Hash Browns – thawed
- 1 cup Shredded Cheese – Mexican Blend or your favorite cheese.
- 5 eggs
- 1/4 cup milk
- 1/2 teaspoon salt
- 1/2 teaspoon pepper
- 2 tablespoon Parmesan – grated

How to Make:

1. Preheat oven to 375 degrees.
2. Take the Crescent Rolls out of the fridge 15 minutes before making.
3. Spray small sheet pan (10×15) with nonstick spray. (TIP: For a deeper style pizza, you can make in a 9×13 casserole dish!)
4. Brown the sausage in a skillet and drain.
5. Spread the rolls on prepared pan.
6. You will have to press and work the dough a little to make sure it covers the pan…pinch the pieces together.
7. Spoon sausage over the crust.
8. Spread the potatoes over the meat.
9. Spread the cheese over the potatoes.
10. Combine eggs, milk, salt, pepper, parmesan together in a separate bowl.
11. Spoon the egg mixture evenly over the cheese.
12. To recap the layering: rolls, meat, potatoes, cheese, egg mixture
13. Bake at 375 degrees for 25-30 minutes or until eggs are set. Oven times vary so check it about halfway through.

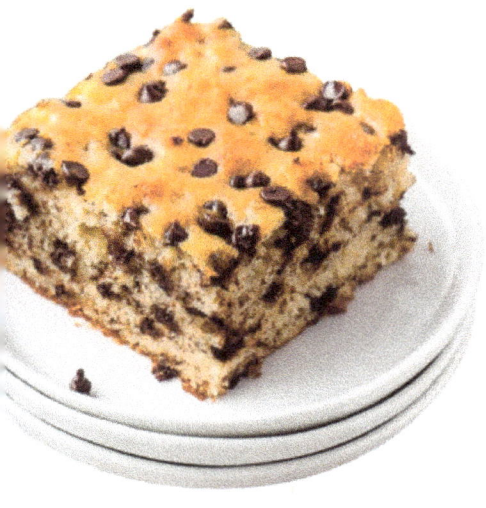

CHOCOLATE CHIP BANANA BARS RECIPE

CHOCOLATE CHIP BANANA BARS RECIPE: My all-time favorite recipe for bananas is this one for Chocolate Chip Banana Bars. Breakfast, lunch, or a snack are all great times to enjoy chocolate chip banana bars! Your entire family will adore them, and they are delicious and filling. They contain a ton of bananas, which I adore. For when we're on the run, I prefer to bake a batch, cut them into squares, and freeze them individually.

My family loves these scrumptious snacks that I've been making for years. I enjoy eating them for breakfast, but they're also great as a snack. They are loaded with bananas, and I make these filling by using whole wheat flour. I understand that adding cinnamon can sound a little unusual, but I urge you to give it a shot.

Ingredients:

- 5 very ripe bananas (about 1 2/3 cup) You may use frozen bananas, of course! When the frozen bananas are ready to be used, thaw them out a little, then peel them and put the bananas in a bowl. Drain the liquid once they have thawed completely, then continue with the preparation.
- 3/4 cup brown sugar
- 1/4 cup oil (any type- I use coconut)
- 1/4 cup milk
- 2 eggs
- 1 3/4 cup flour (I regularly swap out all-purpose flour for whole wheat!)
- 1 tsp baking soda
- 1/2 tsp salt
- 1 tsp cinnamon
- 1 cup mini chocolate chips, divided

How to Make:

1. Pre heat the oven and grease a baking pan.
2. Combine
3. Beat together the butter sugar and eggs. Mix in the other wet ingredients. Stir in the dry ingredients and fold in chocolate chips.
4. Bake
   Pour the batter into the pan, sprinkle chocolate chips on top and bake until cooked through.
   - Heat oven to 350 degrees F. Spray a 15×10.5? Pan with non-stick spray.
   - Peel bananas and mash well. Stir in brown sugar, oil, milk and eggs until combined. Add in dry ingredients and stir. Fold in 1/2 the chocolate chips.
   - Spread the batter into the prepared pan and sprinkle remaining chips on top. Bake 18-22 minutes, until a wooden toothpick inserted in center comes out clean. Cool completely and cut into squares.
   - Makes 24 bars.

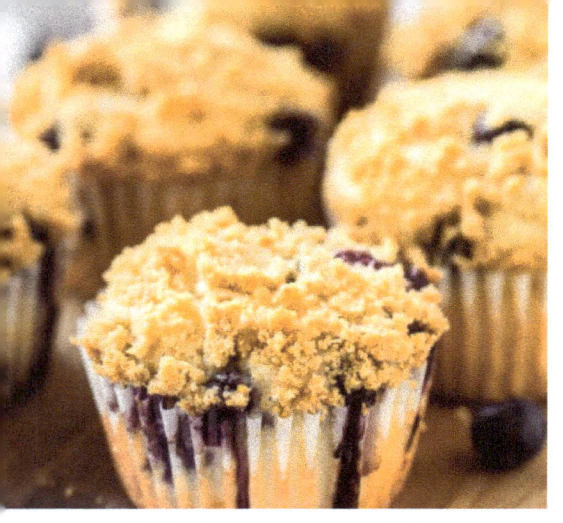

BLUEBERRY MUFFINS RECIPE

Allow me to introduce you to the ultimate blueberry muffin recipe: it's packed with fresh blueberries, enclosed in a light and fluffy muffin batter, and topped with a delightful brown sugar crumble.

It's a simple muffin recipe. In a matter of minutes, you may quickly prepare a homemade muffin mix and topping, pour it into molds, and bake the results.

Spongy muffins these blueberry muffins have the most amazing texture. These are fluffy, moist, and highly addicting since they are made with vegetable oil, sour cream, and buttermilk.

A tasty and delicate crumble topping. These muffins' crumble topping is a straightforward combination of brown sugar, flour, and butter. It is sweet and light, making it the ideal topping for these fluffy muffins.

Ingredients:

- ⅓ cup vegetable oil 67 grams
- 1 cup granulated sugar 200 grams
- ½ cup sour cream 114 grams
- ½ cup buttermilk 114 grams
- 1 large egg 50 grams
- 1 teaspoon pure vanilla extract 4 grams
- 1½ cups all-purpose flour 180 grams, plus 2 teaspoons (5 grams) for the blueberries
- ½ teaspoon kosher salt
- 2 teaspoons baking powder 8 grams
- 1½ cups fresh blueberries 255 grams

How to Make:

1. Make your muffin batter. Whisk together the oil and sugar then whisk in the sour cream, buttermilk, egg and vanilla. Add in the flour, salt and baking powder the whisk again. Finally fold in the blueberries.

2. Make your crumble topping. Prepare the brown sugar topping by mixing brown sugar, butter and flour.

3. Bake. Spoon the batter into the muffin molds, sprinkle on top of the muffins batter and bake for 20-25 mins.

- Preheat oven to 375°F. Grease a 12-count muffin tin or line with paper liners. Set aside.
- Whisk together oil and sugar until fluffy.
- ⅓ cup vegetable oil,1 cup granulated sugar
- Whisk in sour cream,

buttermilk, egg, and vanilla until just combined.

- ½ cup sour cream, ½ cup buttermilk,1 large egg,1 teaspoon pure vanilla extract
- Add in 1½ cups flour, salt, and baking powder and stir. Do not overmix.
- 1½ cups all-purpose flour, ½ teaspoon kosher salt,2 teaspoons baking powder
- Toss fresh blueberries with 2 teaspoons of flour until all the blueberries are coated.
- 1½ cups fresh blueberries
- Add the blueberries into the mixture and gently fold until incorporated, making sure not to break any of the berries.
- Spoon blueberry mixture into the prepared muffin tin until each well is ⅔ full.
- Prepare brown sugar topping by stirring together brown sugar, flour, and melted butter.
- ½ cup brown sugar, ¼ cup all-purpose flour,2 tablespoons unsalted butter
- Sprinkle each muffin with a generous coating of brown sugar topping.
- Bake in oven for 20 to 25 minutes, or until muffins spring back when touched or toothpick comes out clean.
- Let muffins cool on a wire rack.

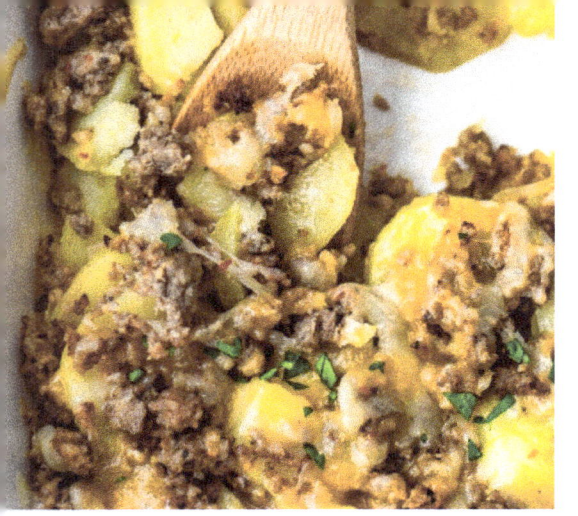

CHEESY SAUSAGE AND POTATOES RECIPE (SAUSAGE BREAKFAST CASSEROLE)

The popular breakfast pairing of potatoes and sausage is delicious. It's very easy to make and so good to eat CHEESY sausage with potatoes. You can quickly prepare a delicious breakfast by preparing this sausage potato casserole in only 30 minutes. For Christmas morning and other special occasions, I especially enjoy making this cheesy sausage breakfast casserole.

Ingredients:

- 2 packages (12 ounces each) JOHNSONVILLE® Original Recipe Breakfast Links
- 1/2 package (20 ounces) frozen roasted potatoes
- 1/2 cup onion, chopped
- 1/2 cup chopped green bell pepper
- 2 cups shredded Cheddar cheese, divided
- 9 large eggs
- 3 cups milk
- 1 tablespoon Dijon mustard
- 1/4 teaspoon salt
- 1/4 teaspoon pepper

How to Make:

1. Cook sausage according to package directions. Cut into 1/4-inch coin-slice pieces.
2. In a large bowl, combine the sausage, potatoes, onion, green pepper and 1-3/4 cups cheese.
3. Spoon into a greased 9x13-inch baking dish.
4. Combine the eggs, milk, mustard, salt and pepper; pour over sausage mixture. Sprinkle with remaining cheese.
5. Bake, uncovered, at 350°F for 45 to 50 minutes or until a knife inserted into the center comes out clean.
6. Let stand 5 minutes before serving.

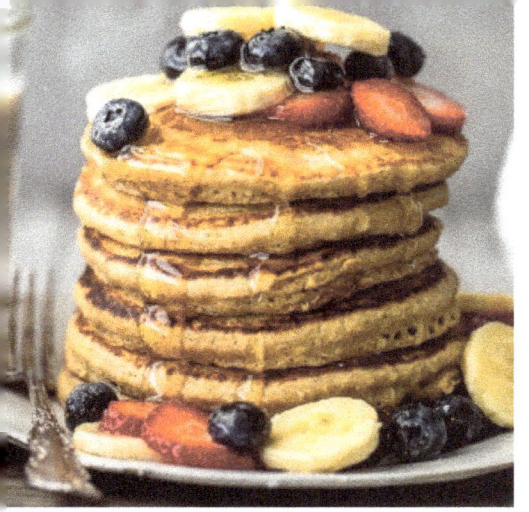

SUPER EASY BANANA PANCAKES (DAIRY FREE PANCAKES MADE IN A BLENDER)

Breakfast may be as easy, delicious, and healthy as making banana pancakes every morning! These vegan pancakes are created without dairy using almond milk, bananas, oats, and a ton of other healthy ingredients. Pancakes that are good for you for breakfast! You're going to adore this simple recipe for banana pancakes.

Pancakes with bananas are the stuff of dreams! (A well-known song has even been composed about them!) Simply put, these HEALTHY banana pancakes taste too delicious to be true. The same mouthwatering flavor of delectable pancakes, but with fantastic ingredient swaps to make them healthy. Consequently, you can eat pancakes for breakfast and feel fine the rest of the day!

Ingredients:

- ½ cup Almond Breeze Almond milk Blended with Real Bananas 114 grams
- 1 ripe banana mashed (plus more for serving)
- 1 large egg 50 grams
- 2 large egg whites 70 grams
- 2 tablespoons honey 44 grams
- 2 cups rolled oats 200 grams
- ½ teaspoon ground cinnamon
- ¾ teaspoon kosher salt
- 1 tablespoon baking powder 12 grams
- 1 teaspoon pure vanilla extract 4 grams

How to Make:

1. Place Almond Breeze Almond milk Blended with Real Bananas, banana, egg and egg whites, honey, oats, cinnamon, salt, baking powder, and vanilla in a high-powered blender.
2. ½ cup Almond Breeze Almond milk Blended with Real Bananas,1 ripe banana,1 large egg,2 large egg whites,2 tablespoons honey,2 cups rolled oats, ½ teaspoon ground cinnamon, ¾ teaspoon kosher salt,1 teaspoon pure vanilla extract,1 tablespoon baking powder
3. Blend until completely smooth.
4. Heat a large griddle or cast-iron skillet over medium heat. Spray with nonstick spray.
5. Use a ⅓-cup measuring cup to

pour batter the onto the griddle in a circle.

6. Cook for 2-3 minutes for the first side, watching for the batter to begin to bubble before flipping.

7. Turn and cook for 1-2 more minutes, or until pancake is browned on both sides to your liking.

8. Top with all the fixings and enjoy!

9. Maple Syrup, Mini Chocolate Chips, Banana Slices, Coconut Flakes, Whipped Cream, Almond Butter, Sliced Strawberries or other berries

SECTION 2:
MAIN DISHES

In a multi-course meal, the main course is the dish that is offered as the main course. It frequently comes after the entrée.

Typically, the largest dish on a menu is the main course. Meat or seafood is frequently the main component. It usually comes after a soup, salad, or appetizer and is frequently followed by dessert.

Dishes we will be looking into:

- Shrimp Diablo
- Broccoli & Cheese Soup
- Chicken Pasta with Ciabatta Croutons
- Italian Mac & Cheese
- Texas Cowboy Hash
- Pork & Veggie Sauté
- Deep Dish Breakfast Pizza
- Deep-Dish Chicken Pot Pie
- Deep-Dish Turkey Pot Pie
- Mandarin Orange Chicken

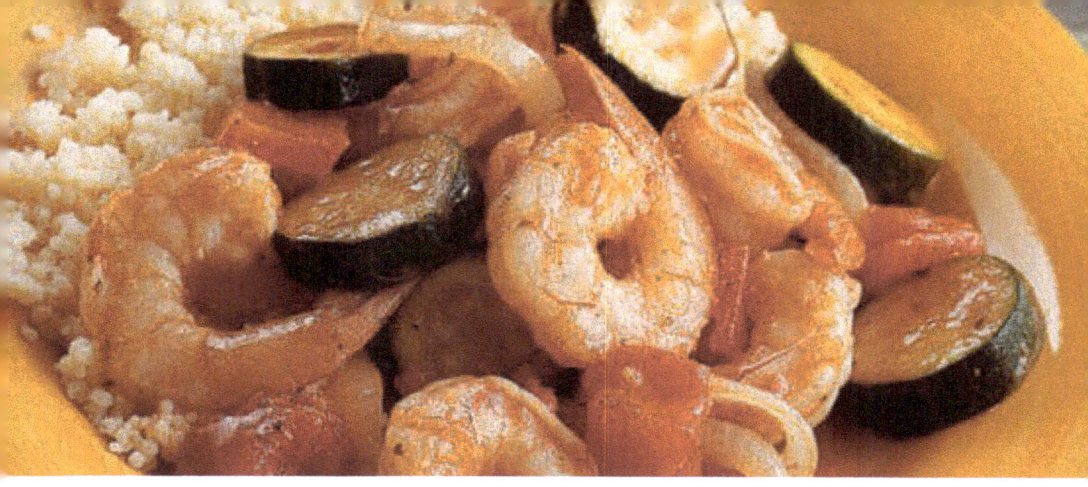

SHRIMP DIABLO

Diablo, which translates to "devil" in Spanish, alludes to the tomato sauce's hot kick that coats the shrimp.

Ingredients:

- 2 tablespoons Land O Lakes® Butter
- 3 medium (3 cups) zucchini, cut into 1/2-inch slices
- 1 medium (1/2 cup) onion, sliced
- 1 teaspoon finely chopped fresh garlic
- 1 (14.5-ounce) can diced tomatoes with Italian herbs
- 1 (12-ounce) package frozen medium cooked shrimp, thawed, drained
- 1/4 teaspoon ground red pepper (cayenne)
- 2 cups hot cooked rice or couscous

How to Make:

1. Melt butter in 10-inch skillet until sizzling; add zucchini, onion and garlic. Cook over medium-high heat, stirring occasionally, 3-4 minutes or until vegetables are crisply tender.

2. Stir in diced tomatoes, shrimp and red pepper. Continue cooking 3-4 minutes or until mixture comes to a full boil. Reduce heat to medium. Cover: cook, stirring occasionally, 6-8 minutes or until shrimp are heated through. Serve over rice.

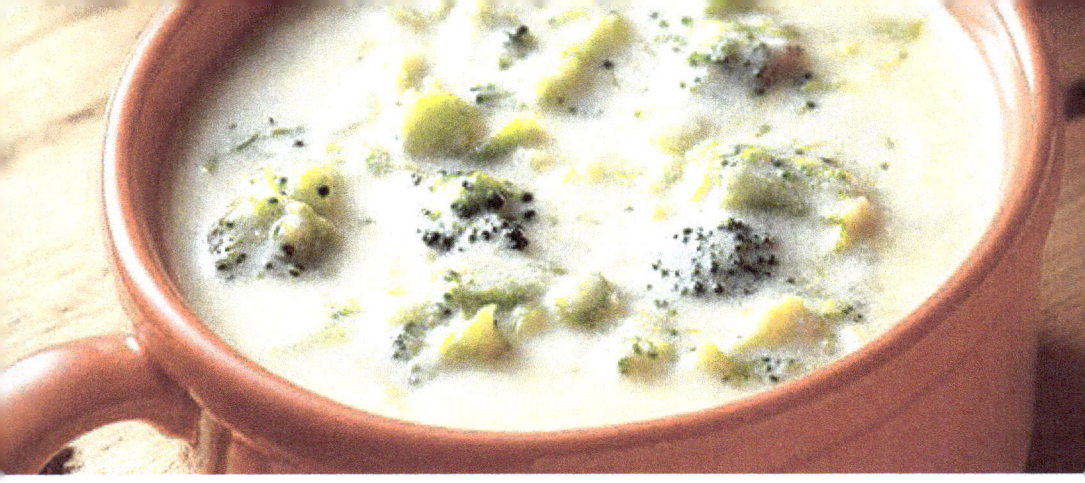

BROCCOLI & CHEESE SOUP

Tonight's dinner should be this quick and simple broccoli cheese soup.

Ingredients:

- 1 (14-ounce) can chicken broth
- 1 (12-ounce) package frozen chopped broccoli
- 1 cup Land O Lakes Fat Free Half & Half
- 2 tablespoons all-purpose flour
- 8 (3/4-ounce) slices Land O Lakes® Deli American, quartered

How to Make:

1. Place chicken broth and broccoli in 2-quart saucepan. Cook over medium-high heat 8-10 minutes or until mixture comes to a boil. Reduce heat to medium. Cook 4-6 minutes or until broccoli is tender.

2. Stir together half & half and flour in bowl until smooth. Slowly add flour mixture to soup, stirring constantly. Continue cooking, stirring occasionally, 2-3 minutes or until mixture comes to a full boil. Boil 1 minute. Reduce heat to low. Stir in cheese until melted.

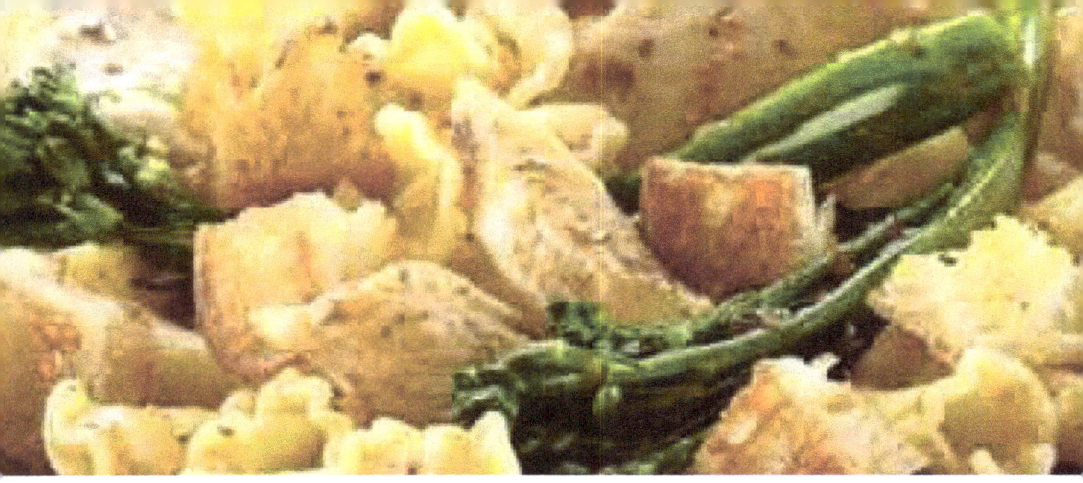

CHICKEN PASTA WITH CIABATTA CROUTONS

The highlight of this dish is the unexpected crunch of the flavored croutons.

Ingredients:

- 2 cups uncooked dried Campanella pasta
- 4 tablespoons Land O Lakes Butter with Olive Oil & Sea Salt
- 2 teaspoons Italian seasoning
- 4 ounces ciabatta bread, cut into 1-inch cubes
- 12 ounces boneless skinless chicken breasts, cut into 1/4-inch-thick strips
- ounces baby broccoli or broccoli florets
- 2 tablespoons fresh lemon juice
- 1 tablespoon finely chopped fresh garlic
- 1/4 teaspoon salt
- 1/4 cup shredded Parmesan cheese, if desired

How to Make:

1. Cook pasta according to package directions. Drain; keep warm.
2. Melt 2 tablespoons Butter with Olive Oil & Sea Salt in 12-inch skillet over medium heat until sizzling. Add Italian seasoning; mix well. Add bread cubes. Cook, stirring occasionally, 3-5 minutes or until bread cubes are slightly crunchy and deep golden brown. Remove bread cubes from skillet.
3. Add chicken to same skillet; cook 4-6 minutes or until lightly browned. Add broccoli and 1 tablespoon lemon juice; continue cooking 8-10 minutes or until broccoli is crisply tender. Remove chicken and broccoli to plate, leaving any sauce in skillet. Cover chicken and broccoli; keep warm.
4. Add remaining 2 tablespoons Butter with Olive Oil & Sea Salt, remaining 1 tablespoon lemon juice, garlic and salt to same skillet. Add pasta; stir to coat pasta with sauce. Stir in bread cubes.
5. Serve cooked chicken and broccoli over pasta. Sprinkle with Parmesan cheese, if desired.

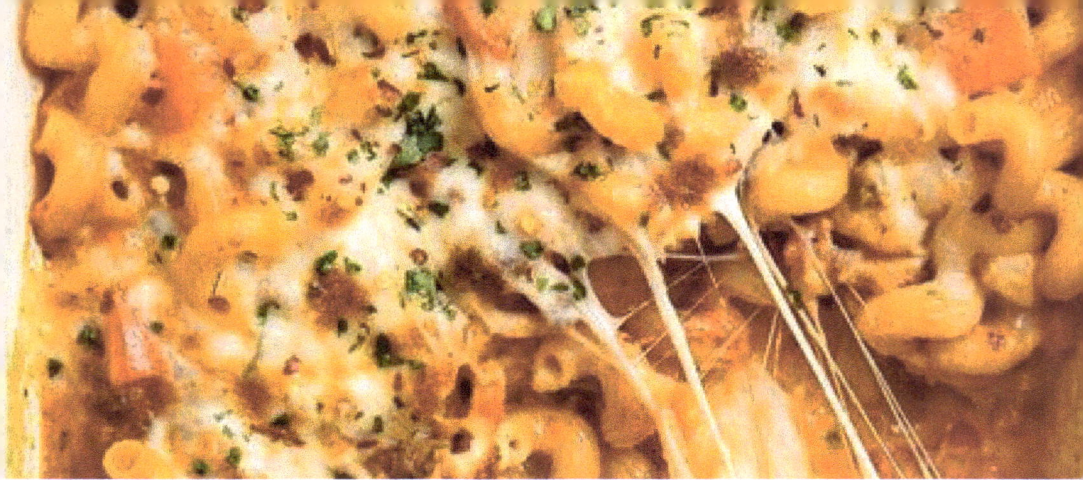

ITALIAN MAC & CHEESE

We've added Italian seasonings to this mac and cheese to give it a unique spin.

Ingredients:

- 8 ounces (2 cups) uncooked penne pasta
- Tablespoons Land O Lakes® Butter
- 1 medium (1/2 cup) onion, chopped
- 2 small zucchinis, halved lengthwise, cut into 1/2-inch chunks
- 3/4 cup sliced roasted red peppers, well drained
- 1/4 cup all-purpose flour
- 1 teaspoon garlic salt
- 1/4 teaspoon pepper
- 2 cups Land O Lakes Half & Half
- 2 teaspoons dried Italian seasoning
- 8-ounce slice Land O Lakes® Provolone Cheese, cubed 1/2 inch
- 1/4 cup Italian-style breadcrumbs

How to Make:

1. Heat oven to 350°f. Spray 3-quart baking dish with no-stick cooking spray; set aside.
2. Cook pasta according to package directions. Drain; keep warm.
3. Meanwhile, melt 4 tablespoons butter in 2-quart heavy saucepan over medium heat until sizzling; add onion. Cook, stirring occasionally, 2-3 minutes or until onion starts to soften. Add zucchini and roasted red peppers; cook 2 minutes. Stir in flour, garlic salt and pepper; continue cooking 1 minute. Gradually stir in half & half and Italian seasoning. Bring to a boil; boil 1 minute. Reduce heat to medium; add cheese. Cook 1-2 minutes or until cheese is melted. Pour mixture over pasta; mix well. Spoon pasta mixture into prepared baking dish.
4. Melt remaining 1 tablespoon butter in 1-quart saucepan. Add breadcrumbs; stir until combined. Sprinkle over pasta mixture. Bake 15-20 minutes or until hot and bubbly and breadcrumbs are browned.

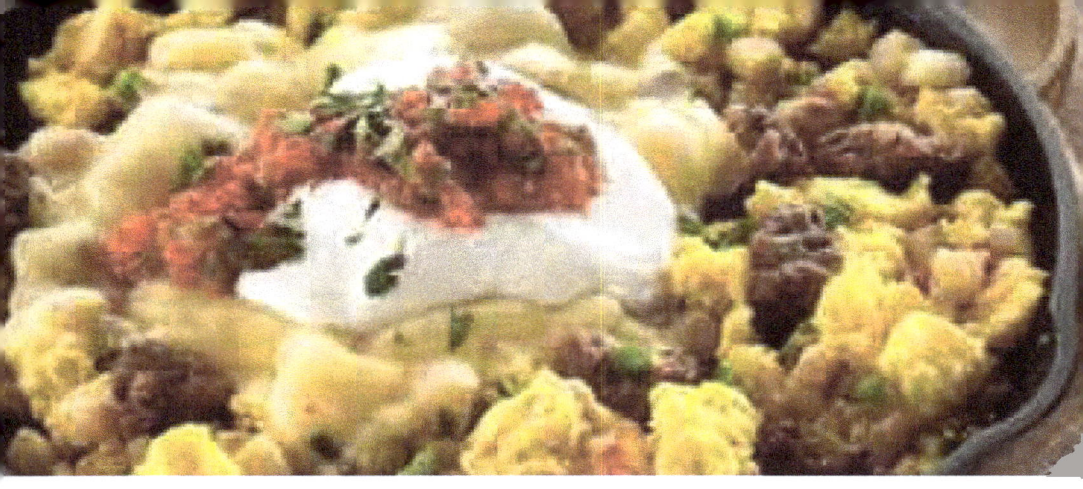

TEXAS COWBOY HASH

Serve this flavorful and filling potato and egg skillet on hectic days when you're short on time.

Ingredients:

- 8 ounces chorizo sausage
- 1 (28-ounce) package frozen diced potatoes with onion and peppers, slightly thawed
- large Land O Lakes Eggs, well beaten
- 2 tablespoons chopped green chiles
- (3/4-ounce) slices Land O Lakes Hot Pepper

How to Make:

1. Cook sausage in 12-inch skillet over medium-heat 6-8 minutes or until no longer pink. Add potatoes; continue cooking, stirring occasionally, 6-8 minutes or until potatoes are tender. Stir in beaten eggs and chiles. Reduce heat to medium. Cook, stirring gently, 1-2 minutes or until eggs are set.
2. Remove from heat, top with cheese slices. Cover: let stand until cheese is melted.
3. Serve with sour cream and salsa, if desired.

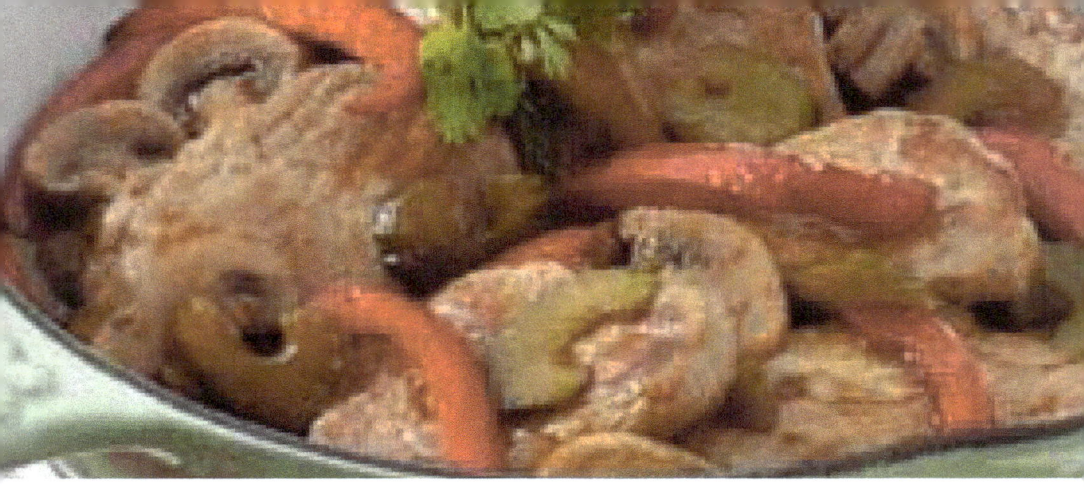

PORK & VEGGIE SAUTE

A fast and delectable skillet supper is made of sliced pork tenderloin and vegetables.

Ingredients:

- 1-pound boneless pork tenderloin
- 2 tablespoons Land O Lakes Butter
- 3 cups sliced fresh vegetables
- 1 teaspoon finely chopped fresh garlic
- 1/4 teaspoon salt

How to Make:

1. Slice pork tenderloin in half lengthwise; then slice crosswise into 1/4-inch-thick slices.

2. Melt butter in 12-inch skillet over medium-high heat until sizzling. Add pork; sauté 4-5 minutes or until pork is browned and cooked through.

3. Add vegetables, garlic and salt; sauté 4-5 minutes or until vegetables are crisply tender.

4. Serve over rice, if desired

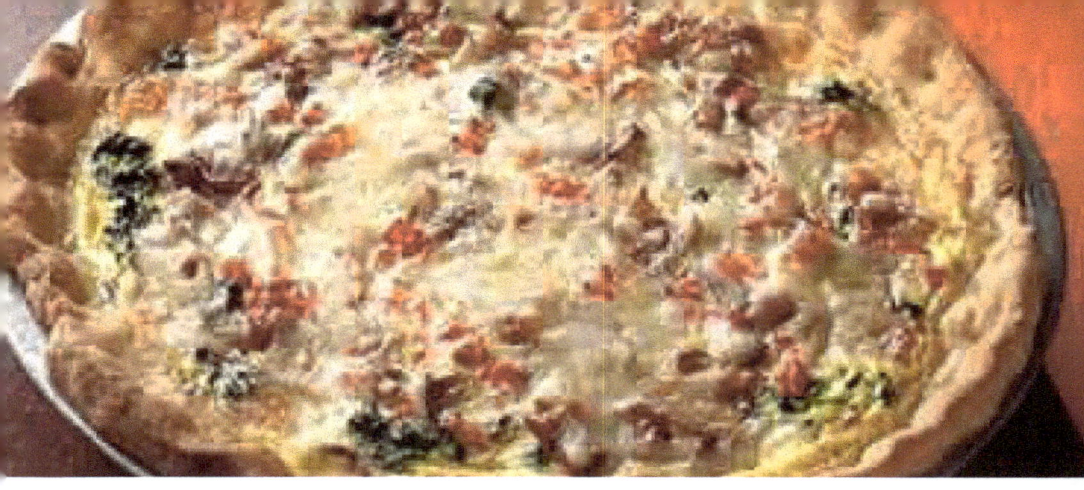

DEEP DISH BREAKFAST PIZZA

The preparation of this filling breakfast is sped up by using chilled pizza crust.

Ingredients:

- 3 tablespoons Land O Lakes Butter
- 2 cups sliced onions
- 1 (10-ounce) can refrigerated pizza crust
- (3/4-ounce) slices Land O Lakes Swiss Cheese, quartered
- 1 (10-ounce) package frozen chopped spinach, thawed, squeezed dry
- 4 slices crisply cooked bacon, crumbled
- 2 tablespoons chopped red bell pepper
- 3 large Land O Lakes Eggs, beaten
- 3/4 cup Land O Lakes Half & Half
- 1/4 teaspoon pepper

How to Make:

1. Heat oven to 350°F. Spray 9-inch pie pan with no-stick cooking spray; set aside.
2. Melt butter in 12-inch nonstick skillet until sizzling; add onions. Cook over medium heat, stirring occasionally, 15-20 minutes or until onions are deep golden brown.
3. Pat or roll pizza crust into 11-inch circle on lightly floured surface. Place into prepared pie pan. Fold under excess dough; pinch edges.
4. Place half of cheese along bottom of crust. Layer cooked onions, spinach, bacon and red pepper over bottom of crust.
5. Combine eggs, half & half and pepper in small bowl; mix well. Pour egg mixture over spinach. Top with remaining cheese pieces. Bake 35-45 minutes or until eggs are set 2 inches from edges. Let stand 10 minutes before serving.

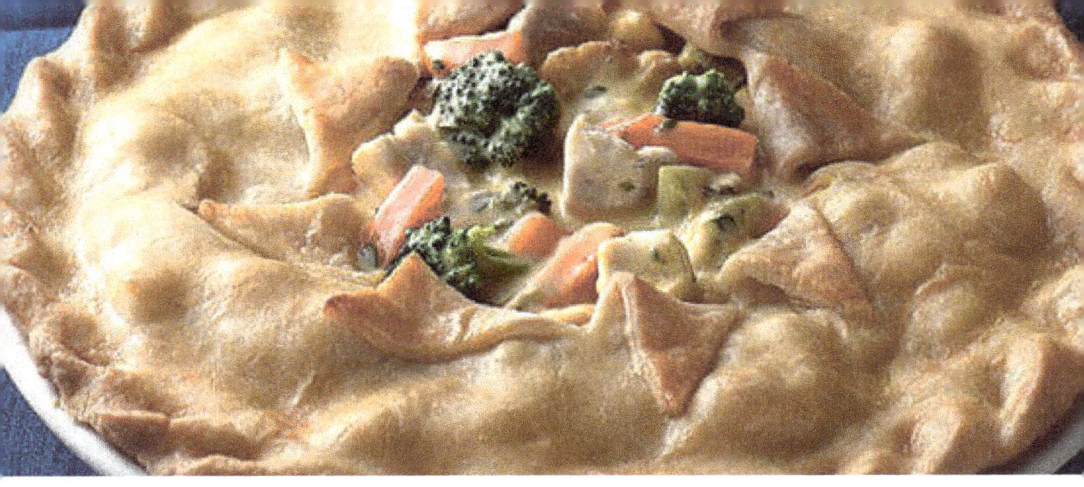

DEEP-DISH CHICKEN POT PIE

On a chilly day, chicken pot pie is the ideal supper. Additionally, chicken leftovers are the ideal ingredient for recipes for chicken pot pies.

Ingredients:

- 2 cups all-purpose flour
- 1/4 teaspoon salt
- 2/3 cup cold Land O Lakes Butter, cut into chunks
- 4 to 6 tablespoons cold water
- 1/4 cup milk
- 1 (10.25-Ounce) can condensed cream of chicken soup
- 2 cups cubed 1-inch cooked chicken or turkey
- 4 (1 cup) ounces shredded Cheddar cheese
- 1 (16-ounce) package frozen vegetable combination (broccoli, cauliflower, carrots)
- 1 1/2 teaspoons fresh thyme leaves
- 1 large Land O Lakes Egg, slightly beaten
- 1 teaspoon water

How to Make:

1. Heat oven to 375°F.
2. Combine flour and salt in bowl; cut in butter with pastry blender or fork until mixture resembles coarse crumbs. Mix in enough cold water with fork until flour is moistened. Divide dough in half. Shape each half into a ball; flatten slightly. Wrap 1 ball in plastic food wrap; refrigerate.
3. Roll out remaining ball of dough on lightly floured surface into 12-inch circle. Fold into quarters. Place dough into ungreased 9 1/2-inch (deep-dish) pie pan; unfold dough, pressing firmly against bottom and sides. Trim crust to 1/2 inch from edge of pan; set aside.
4. Combine milk and soup in bowl; mix well. Add all remaining filling ingredients except egg and 1 teaspoon water. Spoon filling into prepared pie crust.
5. Roll out refrigerated ball of dough on lightly floured surface into 12-inch circle. Cut 3-inch "X" in center of pastry; cut each pastry triangle in half again. Gently fold dough into quarters. Place dough over filling; unfold. Trim, seal and crimp or flute edge. Fold back the 8 points of pastry in center to form an open circle.
6. Combine egg and 1 teaspoon water in bowl; lightly brush crust with egg mixture. Bake 60-70 minutes or until golden brown. Let stand 10 minutes before serving.

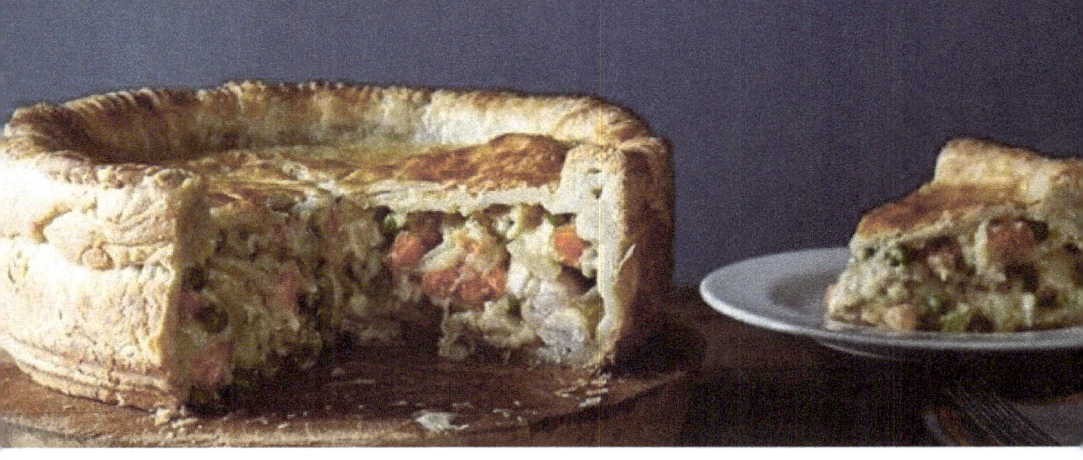

DEEP-DISH TURKEY POT PIE

This unique pot pie recipe is made with turkey and healthy vegetables and has a buttery, flaky crust.

Ingredients:

- 2 cups all-purpose flour
- 1/4 teaspoon salt
- 2/3 cup cold Land O Lakes Butter
- 4 to 6 tablespoons cold water
- 1/4 cup milk
- 1 (10 3/4-ounce) can condensed cream of chicken soup
- 3 cups cubed 1-inch cooked turkey or chicken
- 4 (1 cup) ounces shredded Cheddar Cheese
- 1 (16-ounce) package frozen vegetable combination (broccoli, cauliflower, carrots)
- 1 (16-ounce) can whole potatoes, drained, quartered
- 1/2 teaspoon dried thyme leaves
- 1 large Land O Lakes Egg, slightly beaten
- 1 tablespoon water

How to Make:

1. Heat oven to 375°F.
2. Stir together 2 cups flour and 1/4 teaspoon salt in bowl; cut in 2/3 cup butter with pastry blender or fork until mixture resembles coarse crumbs. Mix in enough cold water with fork until flour is just moistened. Divide dough into thirds. Wrap one-third dough in plastic food wrap; set aside.
3. Roll out remaining two-thirds dough on lightly floured surface into 14-inch circle. Gently fit into 2-quart deep-dish casserole. Trim pastry to 1-inch from edge of casserole; set aside.
4. Combine milk and soup in bowl; mix well. Add all remaining filling ingredients except egg and 1 tablespoon water. Spoon into prepared pie crust.
5. Roll reserved dough on lightly floured surface into 10-inch circle. Cut into 8 (1-inch) strips with sharp knife or pastry wheel. Place 4 strips, 1 inch apart, across filling in casserole. Place remaining 4 strips, 1 inch apart, at right angles to strips already in place: trim strips. Fold trimmed edge of bottom pastry over strips; build up an edge. Crimp or flute edges to seal.
6. Combine egg and 1 tablespoon water in bowl; lightly brush crust with egg mixture. Bake 60-70 minutes or until golden brown. Let stand 10 minutes before serving.

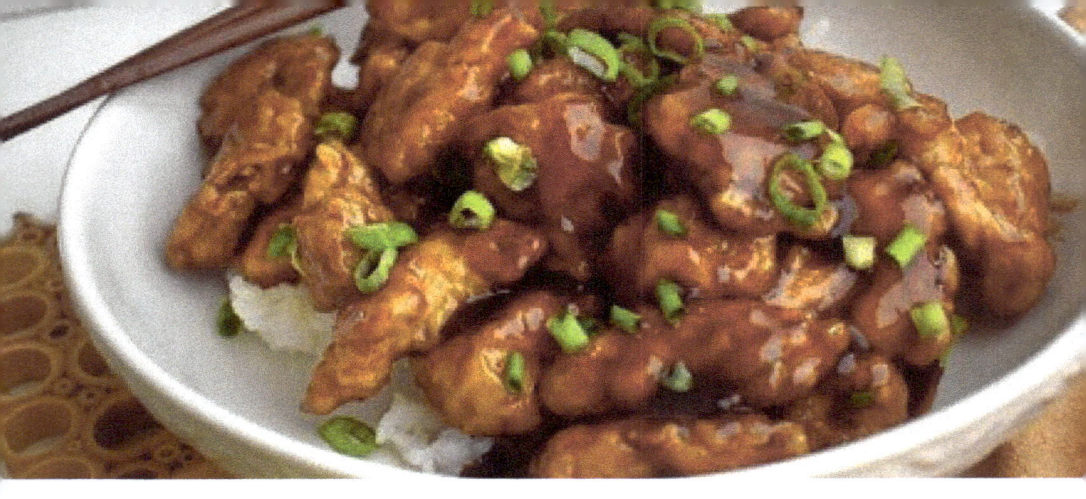

MANDARIN ORANGE CHICKEN

For the ultimate in convenience, use a package of precooked rice to serve with this chicken instead of brown rice, instant rice, or even brown rice.

Ingredients:

1. 2 tablespoons Land O Lakes® Butter
2. 12 chicken drumsticks, skinned
3. 1/2 teaspoon salt
4. 1/4 teaspoon pepper
5. 1/2 cup orange marmalade
6. 1/4 cup chicken broth
7. 2 tablespoons cornstarch
8. 2 tablespoons water
9. 1 (11-ounce) can mandarin orange segments, drained
10. 3 cups hot cooked rice
11. 1 tablespoon sliced green onion

How to Make:

1. Melt butter in 12-inch skillet until sizzling; add chicken drumsticks. Sprinkle with salt and pepper. Cook over medium-high heat, turning once, 4-5 minutes or until chicken is browned.

2. Place chicken into 3 1/2- to 4-quart slow cooker. Combine orange marmalade and chicken broth in small bowl. Pour over chicken. Cover: cook on High heat setting 2-3 hours or on Low heat setting 6-7 hours, or until chicken is tender.

3. Remove chicken to serving platter; cover to keep warm. Strain juices into 1-quart saucepan. Combine cornstarch and water in small bowl; stir into juices. Cook over medium-high heat, stirring constantly, 4-5 minutes or until mixture is thickened. Stir in orange segments. Serve chicken with hot rice and orange sauce. Sprinkle with green onion.

SECTION 3
SNACKS

A snack is a small food serving typically consumed in between meals. Snacks occur in a variety of forms, including items cooked at home from fresh ingredients as well as packaged snack foods and other processed foods.

Snacks are typically made from components that can be found at home with little to no preparation. Snacks are frequently cold cuts, fruits, leftovers, nuts, sandwiches, and sweets. The growth of convenience stores led to a huge increase in the market for packaged snack items. Typically, snack foods are created to be quick, portable, and filling. As a type of convenience food, processed snacks are made to be more enduring, portable, and less perishable than homemade snacks.

SNACKS WE'LL BE LOOKING AT:

1. Apple Cheddar Quesadillas:
2. Cold 'N Creamy Tropical Smoothies
3. Pizza Buns
4. Cinnamon Snack Toss
5. Dragon's Breath Snack Mix

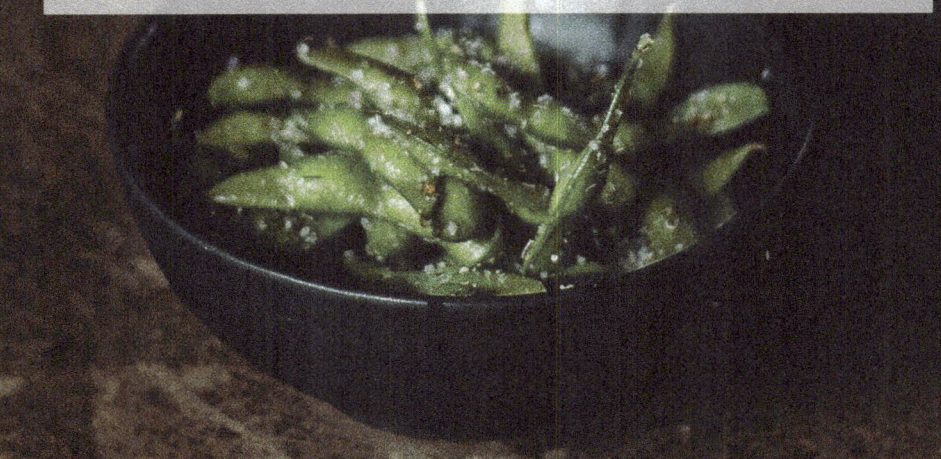

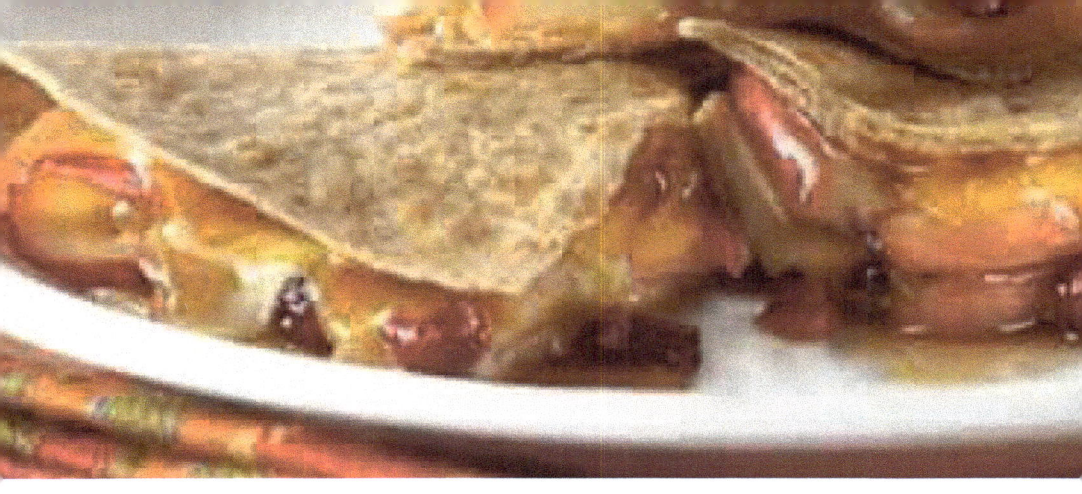

APPLE CHEDDAR QUESADILLAS

Sliced cooked apples, dried cranberries and cheese make a delightful combination for quesadillas.

Ingredients:

- 1/4 cup firmly packed brown sugar
- 1 tablespoon Land O Lakes® Butter
- 1 large (2 cups) tart apple, sliced 1/8 inch
- 1/4 cup sweetened dried cranberries
- 4 (7-inch) low-fat whole-wheat tortillas, warmed
- 4 (3/4-ounce) slices Land O Lakes® Sharp Cheddar American Blend, cut in half diagonally

How to Make:

1. Combine brown sugar and butter in 10-inch skillet. Cook over medium heat, stirring occasionally, 2-3 minutes or until bubbly. Add apple slices; continue cooking 5-8 minutes or until slices are tender. Stir in dried cranberries. Remove from heat.

2. Heat 10-inch skillet or electric griddle over medium heat.

3. Spray 1 side each tortilla with no-stick cooking spray. Layer each, sprayed side down, with 1/4 apple mixture and 2 cheese halves. Fold tortillas in half over mixture.

4. Place 2 quesadillas into skillet. Cook, turning once, 3-5 minutes or until golden brown. (If necessary, wipe out skillet with paper towels.) Repeat with remaining tortillas.

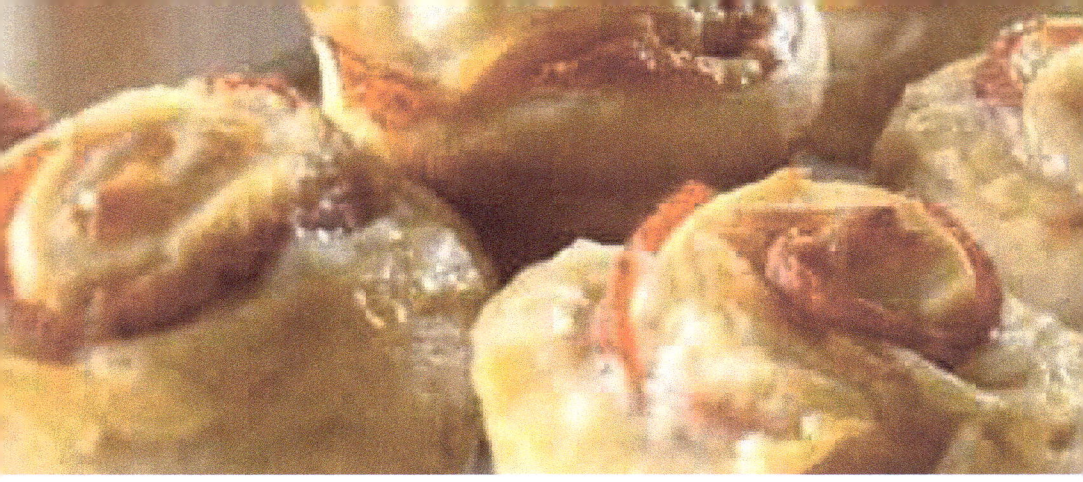

PIZZA BUNS

Ingredients:

- 1 (13.8-ounce) tube refrigerated pizza dough
- 8 (3/4-ounce) slices Land O Lakes® Deli American
- 2 ounces sliced pepperoni

How to Make:

1. Heat oven to 350°F. Grease 12-cup muffin pan; set aside.

2. Pat out dough on lightly floured surface into 15x9-inch rectangle. Place cheese in two rows on long edge of rectangle, leaving 1/2-inch border; top with pepperoni. Roll up dough, starting from cheese edge, into 15-inch log.

3. Slice log into 12 equal pieces. Place each piece into muffin cup. Bake 18-22 minutes or until golden brown and cheese is melted.

4. Remove from oven; run knife around edges of each muffin cup to loosen. Cool in pan 5 minutes; remove to cooling rack.

5. Serve hot or cold with pizza sauce or marinara, if desired. Store refrigerated.

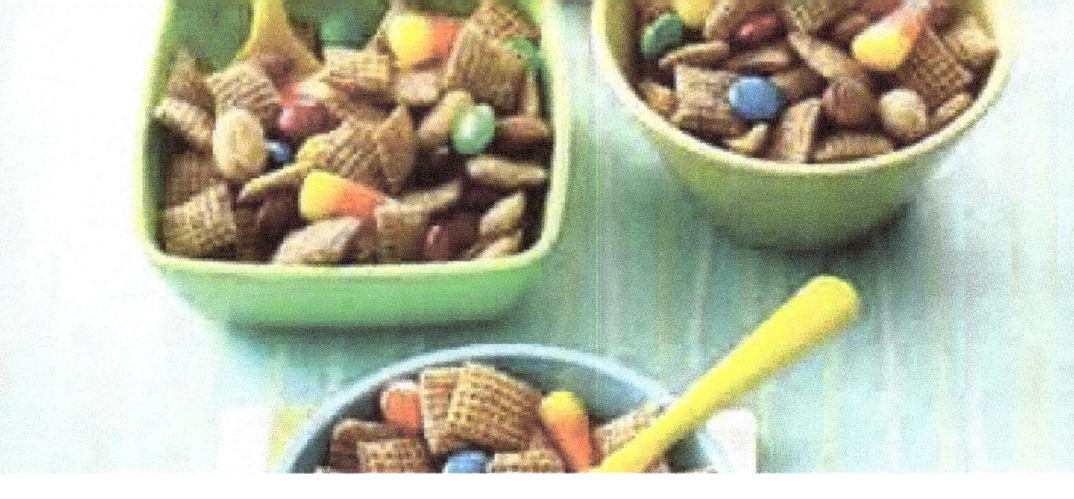

CINNAMON SNACK TOSS

This crunchy caramel snack toss has a dash of cinnamon to enhance it. It's quite simple to make because it's microwaved.

Ingredients:

- 2 cups wheat, corn, or rice cereal
- 1 cup salted peanuts
- 1/2 cup salted whole roasted almonds
- 1 Half Stick (1/4 cup) Land O Lakes® Butter
- 1/3 cup firmly packed brown sugar
- 2 tablespoons light corn syrup
- 1 teaspoon ground cinnamon
- 3/4 cup caramel candy corn
- 3/4 cup candy-coated chocolate pieces or dark chocolate chips

How to Make:

1. Combine cereal, peanuts and almonds in bowl; set aside.
2. Combine butter, brown sugar, corn syrup and cinnamon in small glass measuring cup. Microwave, stirring after each minute, 1-2 minutes or until mixture boils.
3. Pour butter mixture over cereal mixture; stir to coat. Microwave 5 minutes, stirring after each minute. Pour mixture onto waxed paper. Sprinkle with candy corn and chocolate pieces.
4. Cool completely. Store in container with tight-fitting lid.

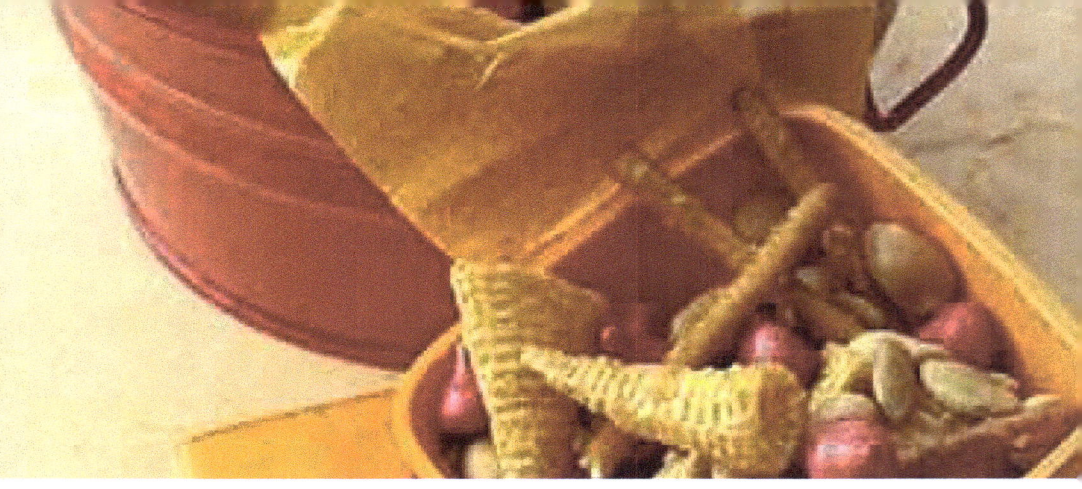

DRAGON'S BREATH SNACK MIX

This vibrant snack mix has flavors of sweet and salty with a touch of spice for an added surprise.

Ingredients:

- cups bugle-shaped corn snacks
- 3 cups pretzel sticks
- 1/2 cup peanuts
- 1/4 cup roasted pumpkin seeds
- 1/3 cup Land O Lakes® Butter, melted
- 2 tablespoons honey
- 1/2 teaspoon red pepper
- 1/2 cup red candy-coated milk chocolate mini kisses or candy-coated chocolate pieces

How to Make:

1. Heat oven to 300°F. Spray 15x10x1-inch baking pan with no-stick cooking spray; set aside.
2. Combine corn snacks, pretzels, peanuts and pumpkin seeds in bowl.
3. Stir together all remaining ingredients except candy-coated kisses in bowl. Pour butter mixture over snack mixture; toss to coat.
4. Spread mixture into prepared pan. Bake, stirring occasionally, 10-12 minutes or until lightly browned. Cool completely. Stir in candy-coated kisses. Store in container with tight-fitting lid

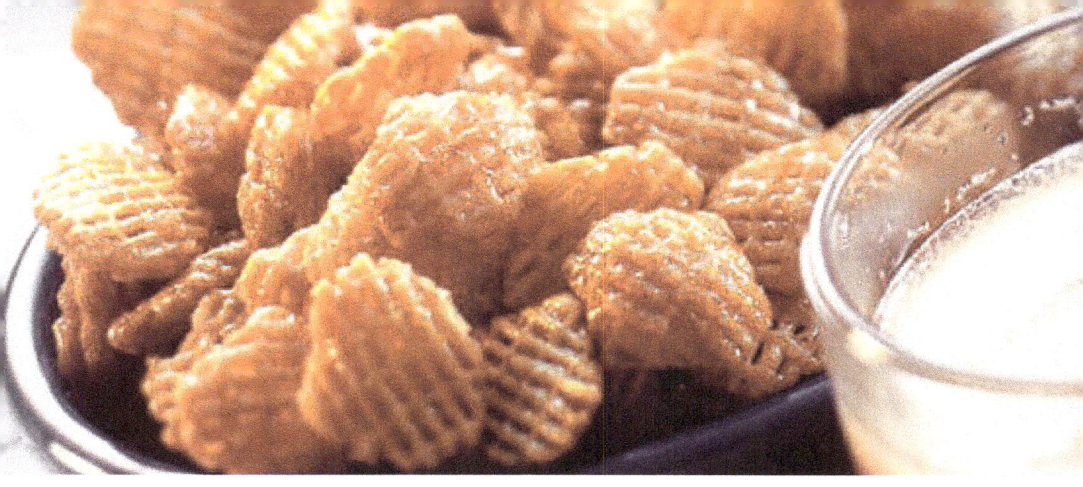

CRISPY GLAZED SNACK MIX

This crunchy, sweet cereal snack mix recipe has a brown sugar coating.

Ingredients:

- 1 (17.9-ounce) box crunchy corn and rice cereal
- 2 cups firmly packed brown sugar
- 1 cup Land O Lakes® Butter
- 1/2 cup light corn syrup
- 1/8 teaspoon salt
- 1/2 teaspoon baking soda

How to Make:

1. Heat oven to 250°F. Spray roasting pan with no-stick cooking spray. Place cereal into prepared pan.

2. Combine brown sugar, butter, corn syrup and salt in 3-quart saucepan. Cook over medium-high heat 8-9 minutes or until mixture comes to a boil. Continue cooking, stirring constantly, 1 minute. Remove from heat. Add baking soda; mix well.

3. Pour syrup mixture over cereal; toss gently until well coated. Bake 40-50 minutes, stirring every 15 minutes, or until coating is set.

4. Spread mixture onto waxed paper. Cool 10 minutes. Break apart. Store in container with tight-fitting lid.

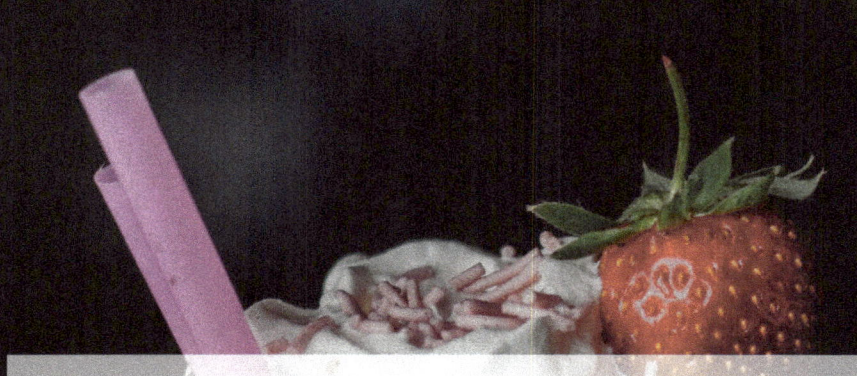

SECTION 4
SMOOTHIES

A smoothie is a drink that is created by blending several ingredients. A liquid basis, such as fruit juice, milk, yogurt, ice cream, or cottage cheese, is a typical component of a smoothie. It is possible to add other components, such as fruits, vegetables, non-dairy milk, ice cubes, whey powder, or nutritional supplements.

SMOOTHIES WE LL BE TREATING:

1. Cold 'n Creamy Tropical Smoothies
2. Blackberry Tea Smoothie
3. Yogurt Parfaits with Granola
4. Lime Cream Cooler
5. Summer Smoothie

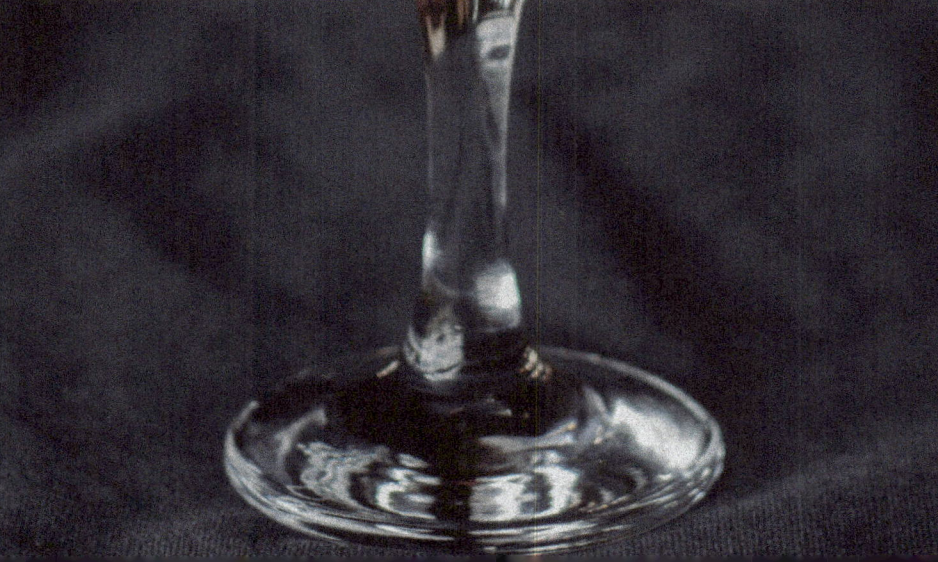

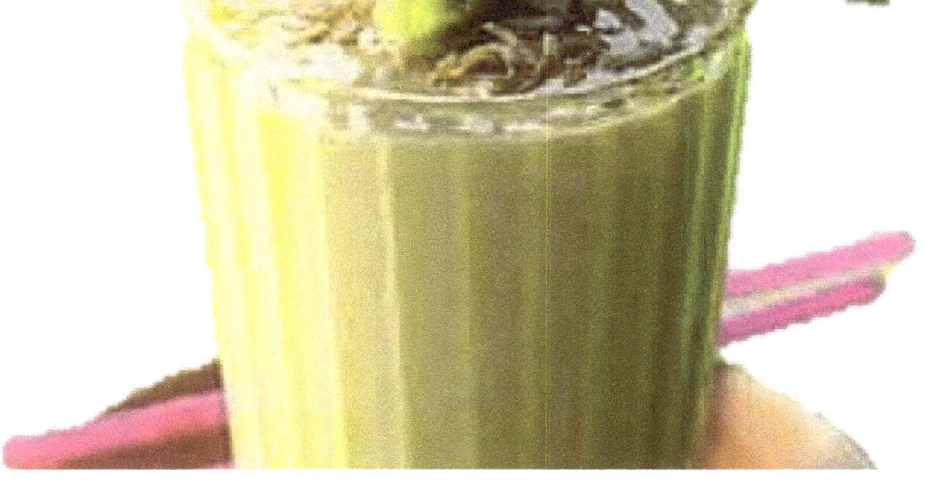

COLD 'N CREAMY TROPICAL SMOOTHIES

This chilled, creamy smoothie is made enticing with half-and-half, yogurt, pineapple, orange, and coconut.

Ingredients:

- 2 cups frozen pineapple chunks
- 1 cup Land O Lakes -Half &Half
- 1 (11-ounce) can mandarin orange segments, drained
- 1 (6-ounce) container coconut-flavored yogurt or your favorite flavor yogurt
- 1 banana or mango, peeled, sliced
- 1 tablespoon fresh lime or lemon juice, if desired

How to Make:

1. Combine all ingredients except toasted coconut in 5-cup blender container. Cover; blend on High until smooth. Pour into 2 (16-ounce) glasses. Sprinkle with toasted coconut, if desired.

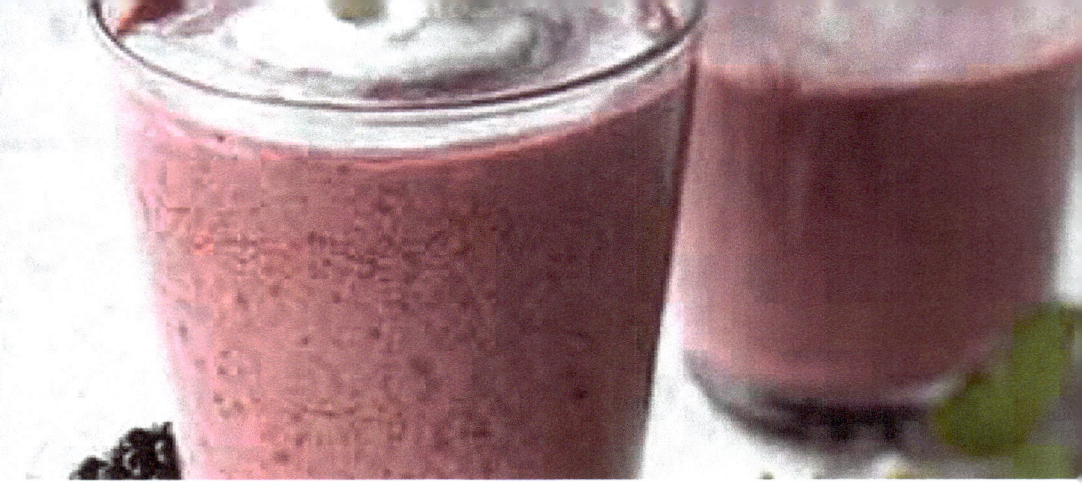

BLACKBERRY TEA SMOOTHIE

In this creamy frozen delicacy, use your preferred frozen berries!

Ingredients:

- 3/4 blackberry tea bags
- 1/2 cup boiling water
- 1 cup Land O Lakes® Half & Half
- 1 cup frozen mixed berries (blackberries, blueberries, strawberries and/or raspberries)
- 1 cup raspberry sherbet
- 2 cups ice cubes
- Land O Lakes® Heavy Whipping Cream, whipped
- Fresh berries, if desired
- 2 tablespoons honey

How to Make:

1. Place tea bags in boiling water; let stand 5 minutes. Squeeze tea bags; remove. Cool tea to room temperature.
2. Combine tea and all remaining smoothie ingredients in 5-cup blender container. Cover; process 30-60 seconds or until smooth. Pour into individual glasses. Garnish with whipped cream and fresh berries, if desired.

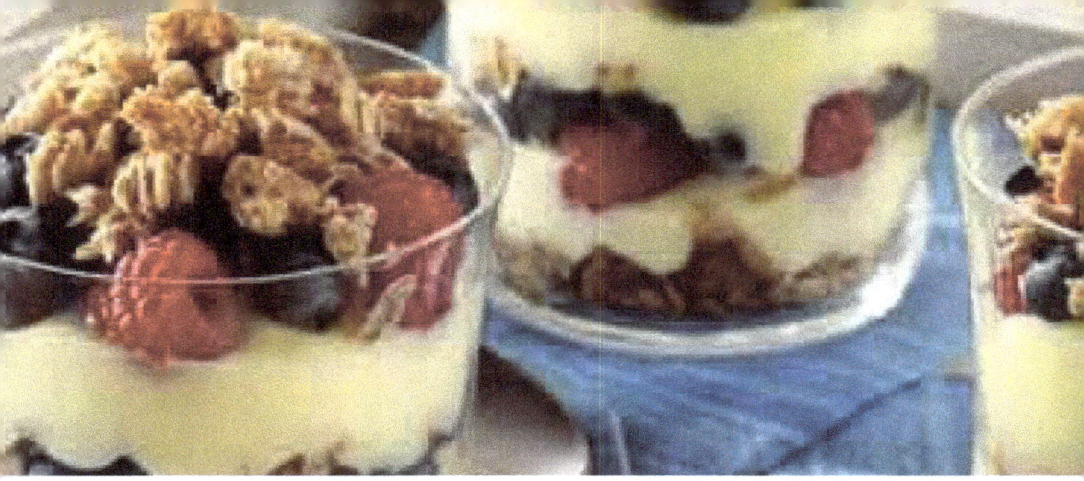

YOGURT PARFAITS WITH GRANOLA

The parfaits are simple to make, and kids will like them for breakfast or as a nutritious snack.

Ingredients:

- 1/2 cup uncooked old-fashioned or quick-cooking oats
- 1/2 cup coarsely chopped graham crackers
- 3 tablespoons Land O Lakes® Cinnamon Sugar Butter Spread
- 2 cups vanilla yogurt
- 2 cups fresh fruit

How to Make:

1. Heat oven to 350°F.
2. Combine all granola ingredients in bowl; stir well to combine. Spread into lightly greased 9-inch square baking pan. Bake, stirring once, 11-12 minutes or until golden brown. Cool completely; break apart.
3. Layer ingredients starting with 1 tablespoon granola, 1/4 cup yogurt and 1/4 cup fruit; repeat layers ending with granola.
4. Serve immediately or cover each with plastic food wrap. Refrigerate up to 2 hours.

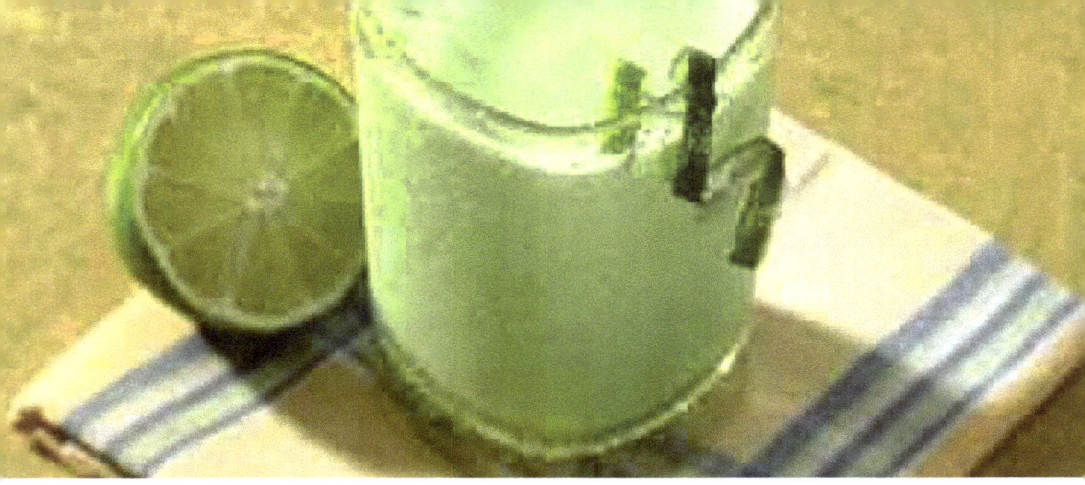

LIME CREAM COOLER

A creamy, cool punch recipe is ideal as a drink at a summer party or as a cool treat on a hot summer day.

Ingredients:

- 1 quart (4 cups) vanilla ice cream, slightly softened
- 1 quart (4 cups) lime sherbet, slightly softened
- 4 cups Land O Lakes® Fat Free Half & Half
- 1 (6-ounce) can froze lemonade concentrate
- 1 (6-ounce) can froze limeade concentrate
- 2 cups water
- 4 cups ginger ale

How to Make:

1. Stir together ice cream, sherbet, and fat free half & half in large punch bowl.
2. Stir together lemonade concentrate, limeade concentrate and water in 1-quart pitcher. Pour over ice cream mixture. Add ginger ale; stir until slightly mixed.

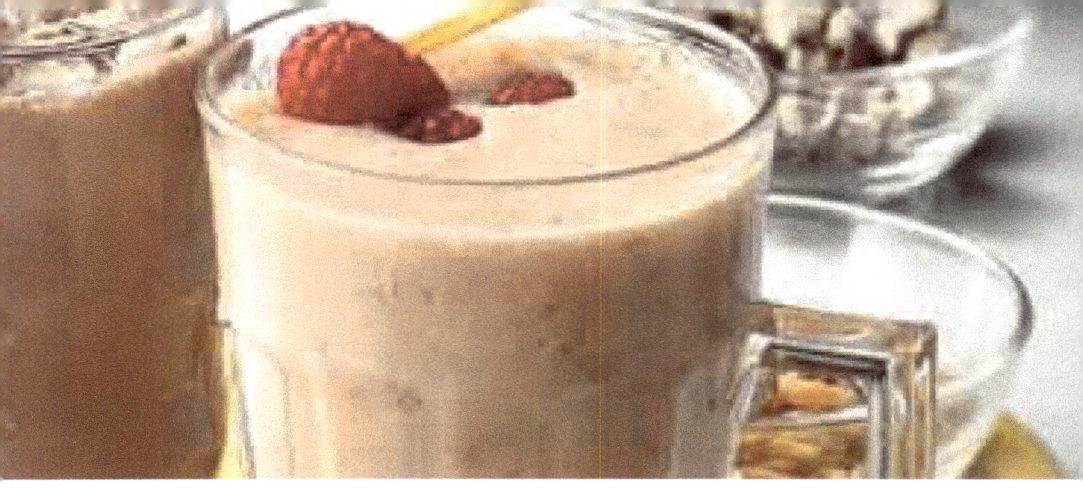

SUMMER SMOOTHIE

This vitamin-rich beverage is made from ripe summer fruits.

Ingredients:

- 1 1/2 cups low fat frozen peach yogurt
- 1 cup chopped fresh cantaloupe
- 1/2 cup fresh raspberries
- 1/2 cup peeled, chopped fresh mango
- 1/4 cup Land O Lakes® Fat Free Half & Half

How to Make:

1. Combine all smoothie ingredients in 5-cup blender container. Cover; blend until smooth.
2. Stir in any one or more stir-ins, if desired. Serve smoothies with spoons.

SECTION 5
DESSERTS

A meal's final course is usually dessert. The course comprises of sweet treats like candies and perhaps a drink like dessert wine or liqueur. There isn't a customary dessert dish to end a dinner in various parts of the world.

Some Desserts we'll be looking at:

1. Apple Ginger Pie
2. Caramel Apple Upside-Down Cake
3. Candy Cane Dessert Squares
4. Chocolate Cream Macaroon Tarts
5. Pineapple Delight Cheesecake

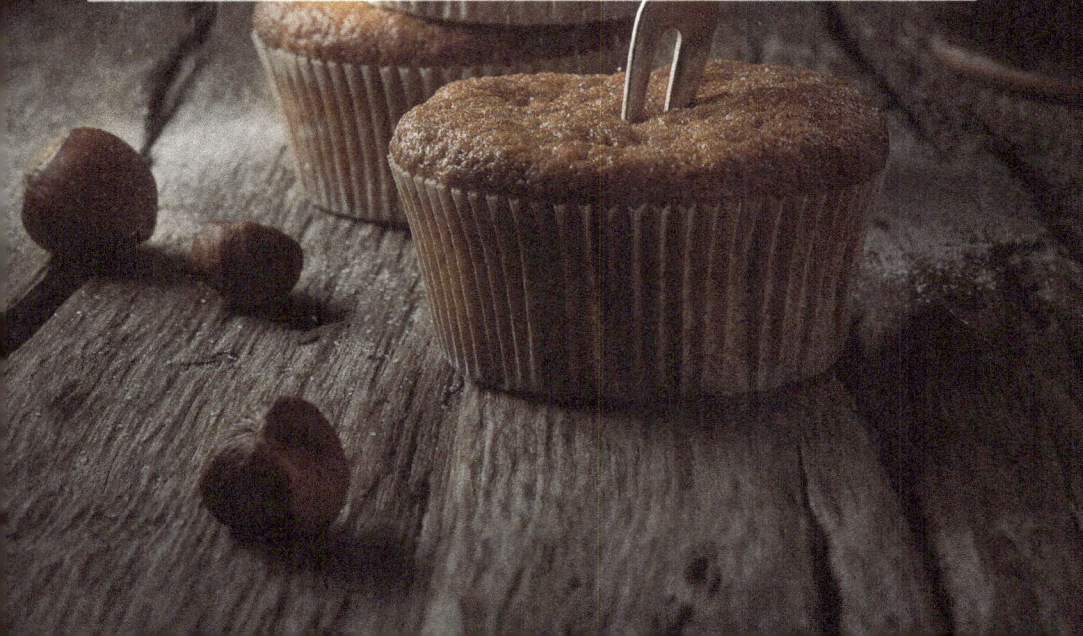

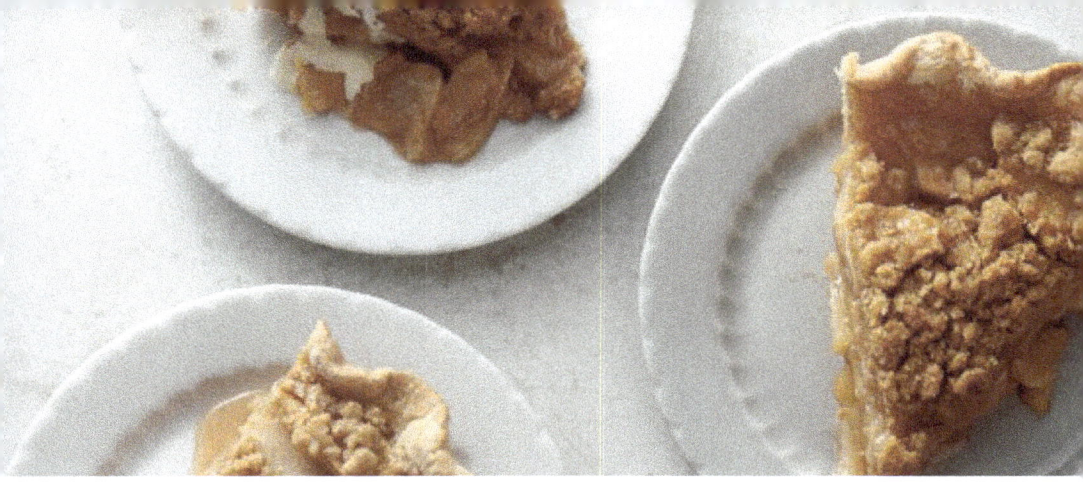

APPLE GINGER PIE

For hassle-free entertaining, this decadent tropical cheesecake recipe can be prepared in advance

Ingredients:

- 1 cup all-purpose flour
- 1/2 teaspoon sugar
- 1/8 teaspoon salt
- 1/8 teaspoon ground cinnamon
- 1/8 teaspoon ground ginger
- 1/3 cup cold Land O Lakes® Butter, cut into chunks
- 2 to 3 tablespoons cold water
- 1/2 cup sugar
- 1/4 cup firmly packed brown sugar
- 1/4 cup all-purpose flour
- 1/2 teaspoon ground cinnamon
- 1/2 teaspoon ground ginger
- medium (6 cups) tart cooking apples, peeled, sliced 1/4-inch
- 1/2 cup all-purpose flour
- 1/3 cup firmly packed brown sugar
- 1/2 teaspoon ground ginger
- 1/4 cup Land O Lakes® Butter, softened
- Ice cream, if desired

How to Make:

1. Heat oven to 400°F.
2. Combine all crust ingredients except 1/3 cup butter and water in bowl. Cut in 1/3 cup butter with pastry blender or fork until mixture resembles coarse crumbs. Stir in enough water with fork just until moistened.
3. Shape dough into a ball; flatten slightly. Roll out on lightly floured surface into 12-inch circle. Fold into quarters. Place dough into ungreased 9-inch pie pan; unfold dough, pressing firmly against bottom and sides. Crimp or flute edge. Refrigerate while preparing filling.
4. Combine all filling ingredients except apples in bowl. Add apples; toss lightly to coat. Spoon apple mixture into prepared crust.
5. Combine all streusel ingredients except 1/4 cup butter in bowl. Cut in 1/4 cup butter using pastry blender or fork until mixture resembles coarse crumbs: sprinkle evenly over filling. Cover edge of crust with 2-inch strip aluminum foil.
6. Bake 30 minutes; remove foil. Continue baking 10-12 minutes or until crust is lightly browned and juice begins to bubble through streusel. Cool 1 hour.
7. Serve warm with ice cream, if desired.

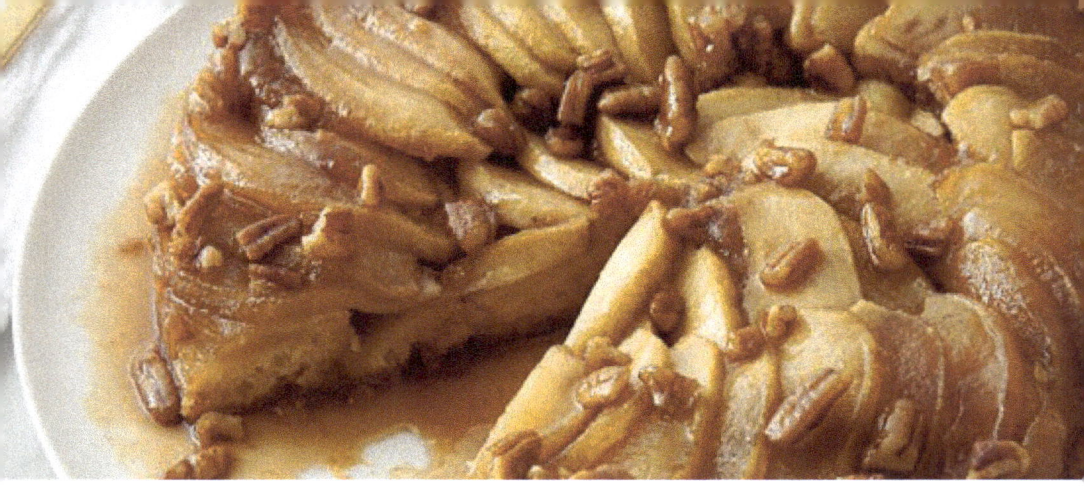

CARAMEL APPLE UPSIDE-DOWN CAKE

This old-fashioned dessert is a classic for a reason. Brown sugar and butter melt and bake into a sweet caramel sauce that tops the cake when flipped after baking.

Ingredients:

TOPPING
- 1 cup firmly packed brown sugar
- tablespoons cold Land O Lakes® Butter, cut into chunks
- 1/4 cup chopped pecans
- 2 large Granny Smith apples, peeled, cored, thinly sliced

CAKE
- 1 1/2 cups all-purpose flour
- 1 teaspoon baking powder
- 1/2 teaspoon salt
- 2/3 cup firmly packed brown sugar
- 1/3 cup Land O Lakes® Butter, softened
- 1 large Land O Lakes® Egg
- 1 teaspoon vanilla extract
- 1/2 cup milk

How to Make:

1. Heat oven to 350°F. Grease 9-inch round cake pan; set aside.
2. Place 1 cup brown sugar into bowl; cut in 6 tablespoons butter with pastry blender or fork until mixture resembles coarse crumbs. Stir in pecans. Press onto bottom of prepared pan. Arrange apple slices on top. Set aside.
   - Tip: Layering Apples helps get more in the pan and looks better
3. Combine flour, baking powder and salt in bowl. Set aside.
4. Combine 2/3 cup brown sugar and 1/3 cup butter in another bowl. Beat at medium speed, scraping bowl often, until creamy. Add egg and vanilla; continue beating until smooth. Add flour mixture alternately with milk until well mixed. Spoon batter over apple layer; spread evenly.
5. Tip: Spooning Batter into Pan
6. Bake 35-40 minutes or until toothpick inserted in center comes out clean. Cool 5 minutes; invert onto serving plate. Serve warm or cool.

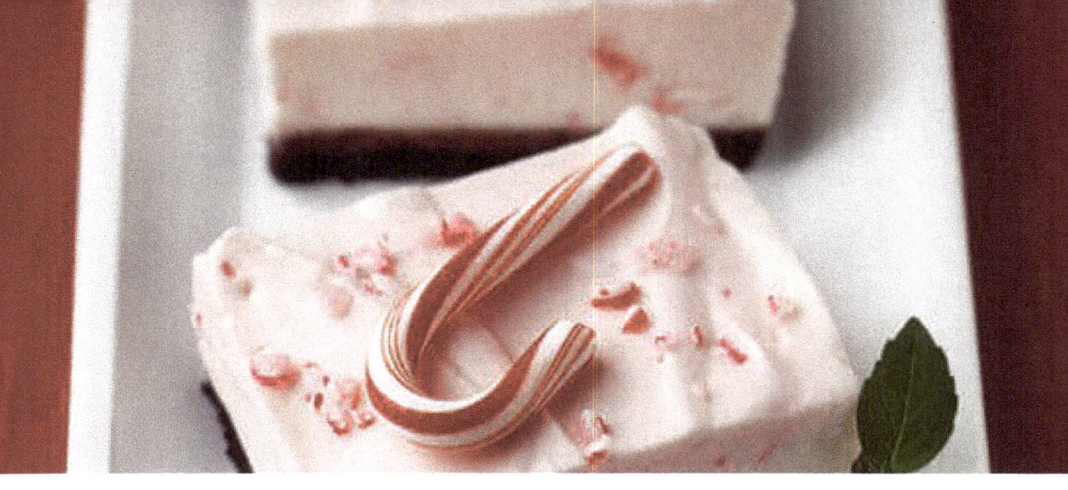

CANDY CANE DESSERT SQUARES

Suitable for a large holiday dinner party, this recipe for a candy cane dessert serves a lot of people.

Ingredients:

CRUST
- 36 (2 cups) chocolate wafer cookies, finely crushed
- 1/2 cup Land O Lakes® Butter, melted
- 3 tablespoons sugar

GANACHE
- 1 cup semi-sweet chocolate chips
- 2/3 cup Land O Lakes® Heavy Whipping Cream

FILLING
- 1 cup powdered sugar
- 2 (8-ounce) packages cream cheese, softened
- 2 teaspoons peppermint extract
- 1 1/2 cups Land O Lakes® Heavy Whipping Cream, whipped
- 2/3 cup coarsely crushed red or green hard peppermint candies

How to Make:

1. Heat oven to 325°F.
2. Combine all crust ingredients in bowl. Press onto bottom of ungreased 13x9-inch baking pan. Bake 10 minutes. Cool completely. Set aside.
3. Melt chocolate chips and 2/3 cup whipping cream in 1-quart saucepan over low heat, stirring occasionally, 4-5 minutes or until smooth. Spread evenly over crust. Place in freezer at least 10 minutes while making filling.
4. Combine powdered sugar, cream cheese and peppermint extract in bowl. Beat at low speed, scraping bowl often, until smooth and creamy. Gently stir in whipped cream and crushed candies. Spread evenly over ganache layer. Sprinkle with additional crushed candy, if desired. Cover; freeze 4 hours or overnight.
5. Cut into squares. Top each serving with small candy cane, if desired. Serve frozen or refrigerated. Store frozen.

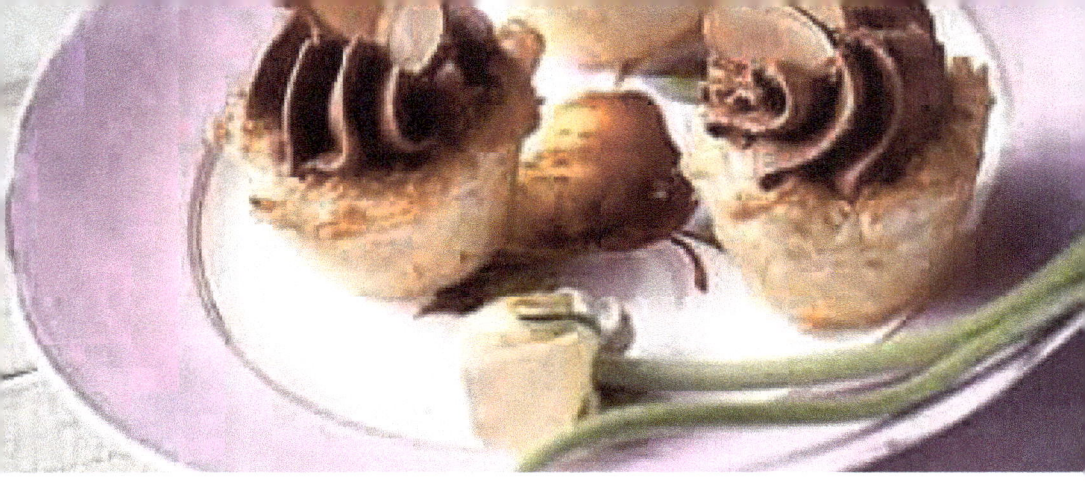

CHOCOLATE CREAM MACAROON TARTS

The filling for this easy macaroon tart recipe is a luscious chocolate buttercream.

Ingredients:

CRUST
- 1 1/2 cups sweetened flaked coconut
- 1/4 cup sugar
- 2 large Land O Lakes® Eggs (whites only)

FILLING
- 1/4 cup Land O Lakes® Butter, softened
- 1 2/3 cups powdered sugar
- 2 tablespoons Land O Lakes® Heavy Whipping Cream
- 1/4 teaspoon almond extract
- 1 tablespoon light corn syrup
- 2 (1-ounce) squares unsweetened baking chocolate, melted, cooled
- 1/4 cup sliced almonds, toasted

How to Make:

1. Heat oven to 350°F.
2. Combine coconut, sugar and egg whites in bowl; mix well.
3. Spray 16 mini muffin pan cups with no-stick cooking spray. Press 1 tablespoon coconut mixture on bottom and up sides of each cup. Place muffin pans onto baking sheet.
4. Bake 13-16 minutes or until tarts begin to brown. Cool slightly. Remove from pans. Cool completely.
5. Beat butter in another bowl at medium speed until creamy. Continue beating, gradually adding powdered sugar alternately with whipping cream and almond extract and scraping bowl often, until light and fluffy. Add corn syrup; mix well. Stir in melted chocolate.
6. Place filling into pastry bag fitted with star tip. Pipe filling evenly into coconut crusts. Garnish with almonds.

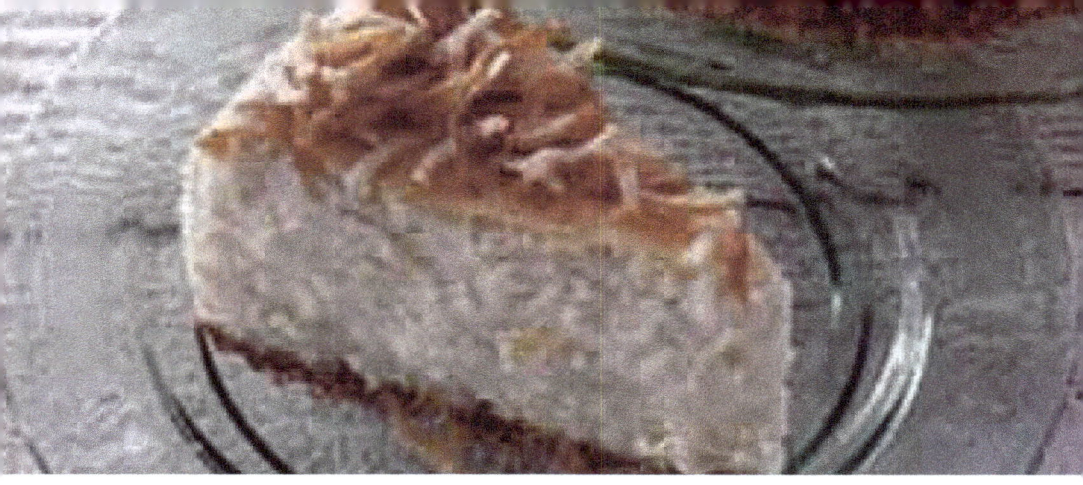

PINEAPPLE DELIGHT CHEESECAKE FOR PASSOVER

For hassle-free entertaining, this decadent tropical cheesecake recipe can be prepared in advance.

Ingredients:

CRUST
- 1/3 cup matzo meal
- 1/3 cup potato starch
- 1/4 cup firmly packed brown sugar
- 1/4 cup cold Land O Lakes® Butter

FILLING
- 1 cup sugar
- 4 (8-ounce) packages cream cheese, softened
- 4 large Land O Lakes® Eggs
- 1 cup sour cream
- 1 cup sweetened flaked coconut
- 1 (20-ounce) can crushed pineapple in juice, well-drained

TOPPING
- 1/2 cup sweetened flaked coconut, toasted
- 1 teaspoon freshly grated orange zest

How to Make:

1. Heat oven to 325°F.
2. Place all crust ingredients except butter in food processor bowl fitted with metal blade. Cover: process 30-60 seconds or until ingredients are mixed. Add butter, process just until mixed. Press crumb mixture evenly onto bottom of ungreased 9-inch springform pan. Bake 10 minutes. Cool completely.
3. Combine sugar and cream cheese in bowl. Beat at medium speed, scraping bowl often, 3-4 minutes or until creamy. Continue beating, adding eggs one at a time and beating well after each addition. Add sour cream, 1 cup coconut and drained pineapple. Continue beating, scraping bowl often, until well mixed.
4. Spoon cream cheese mixture into prepared crust. Bake 70-90 minutes or until set 2 inches from edge of pan. Sprinkle top with 1/4 cup toasted coconut. Turn off oven; leave cheesecake in oven 2 hours.
5. Loosen sides of cheesecake from pan by running knife around inside of pan. Cover; refrigerate 8 hours or overnight. Sprinkle with remaining toasted coconut and orange zest.

Appendix

The last thing I'm going to leave you with is a cooking conversion chart. This is to help you out if you need to convert measurements, or anything of the like so that you can enjoy the recipes from anywhere in the world.

Dry Weights

Ounces	Tablespoons	Cups	Grams	Pounds
½ ounce	1 tablespoon	1/16 cup	15 grams	---
1 ounce	2 tablespoons	1/8 cup	28 grams	---
2 ounces	4 tablespoons	¼ cup	57 grams	---
3 ounces	6 tablespoons	1/3 cup	85 grams	---
4 ounces	8 tablespoons	½ cup	115 grams	¼ pound
8 ounces	16 tablespoons	1 cup	227 grams	½ pound
12 ounces	24 tablespoons	1 ½ cups	340 grams	¾ pound
16 ounces	32 tablespoons	2 cups	455 grams	1 pound

Oven Temp

Celcius	240	230	220	200	190	180	170	150	140	120
Farenheit	475	450	425	400	375	350	325	300	275	250

Liquid Conversions

- "One gallon = 4 quarts, 8 pints, 16 cups, 128 fluid ounces, 3.8 liters

- One quart = 2 pints, 4 cups, 32 fluid ounces, 946 milliliters

- One pint = 2 cups, 16 fluid ounces, 470 milliliters

- One cup = 16 tablespoons, 8 fluid ounces, 240 milliliters

- ¼ cup = 4 tablespoons, 2 fluid ounces, 12 teaspoons, 60 milliliters"

Liquid Volumes

Ounces	Teaspoons	Tablespoons	Milliliters	Cups	Pints	Quarts
1	6	2	30	1/8	--	--
2	12	4	60	¼	--	--
2 2/3	16	5	80	1/3	--	--
4	24	8	120	½	--	--
5 1/3	32	11	160	2/3	--	--
6	36	12	177	¾	--	--
8	48	16	240	1	½	¼
16	96	32	470	2	1	½
32	192	64	950	4	2	1

- 1 tsp = 5mL
- 1 tbsp = 15 mL
- Dash = 1/16 tsp
- Pinch = 1/8 tsp

Conclusion

You've reached the end of *Cooking With Sgt Perez*. I hope that you enjoy all of the recipes, and find them easy and enjoyable to make. I hope that the cookbook is something that you use over and over again, and enjoy the recipes. Lastly, I would like to ask that if you have found the book helpful in any way, a positive review on Amazon or with Barnes & Noble is always helpful.

THANK YOU & ENJOY!

No matter how busy your life is, you can always find time to cook a delicious and nutritious meal. With a little planning and the right ingredients, you can make a meal that will not only taste good but will also help you stay healthy and fit. We hope that these recipes have inspired you to get in the kitchen and start cooking for yourself. If you're looking for some quick and easy meal ideas that are perfect for a busy, tactical lifestyle, then cooking with Sgt. Perez is the way to go. My recipes are simple but delicious, and they can be easily tailored to your own personal preferences. Plus, my tips on food storage and preparation will help you save time and hassle in the kitchen.

In conclusion, the book is a great way to improve your health and is a great way to make quick meals that are nutritious and delicious. With a little bit of planning, you can make sure that you always have something healthy and tasty to eat, no matter how busy your life gets.

Thanks for reading!

CHECK OUT

THESE OTHER COOKBOOKS FROM SGT PEREZ

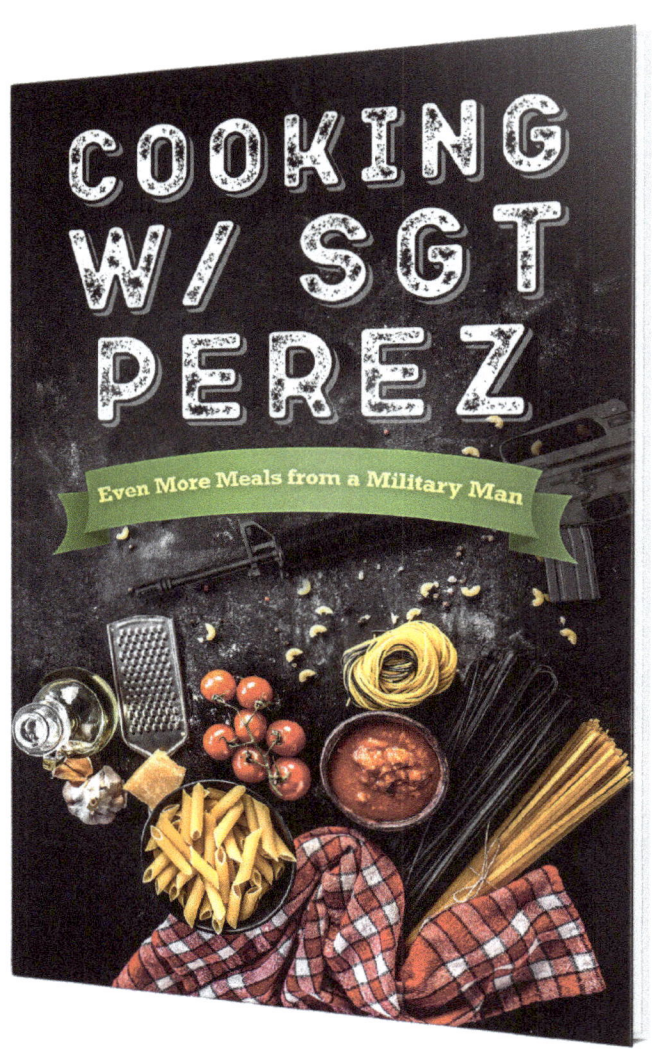

CONTINUING THE JOURNEY OF DELICIOUS AND QUICK CULINARY CREATIONS, "COOKING WITH SGT PEREZ: EVEN MORE MEALS FROM A MILITARY MAN" BRINGS AN ENTIRELY NEW SET OF RECIPES TAILORED FOR THOSE WITH A DYNAMIC LIFESTYLE. IF YOU'VE EVER FELT THE CONSTRAINTS OF A BUSTLING SCHEDULE OR THE DEMANDING NATURE OF TACTICAL PROFESSIONS LIKE THE MILITARY OR LAW ENFORCEMENT, AND YEARN FOR VARIETY AND NUTRITION IN YOUR MEALS, THIS SEQUEL IS CRAFTED JUST FOR YOU. THIS BOOK IS A TESTAMENT TO THE BELIEF THAT EVEN IN THE WHIRLWIND OF OUR DAILY LIVES, PREPARING AND ENJOYING WHOLESOME, TASTY FOOD SHOULD NEVER BE A COMPROMISE.

IN THIS SECOND INSTALLMENT, SGT PEREZ GOES BEYOND THE BASICS, INTRODUCING RECIPES THAT CATER TO A WIDE ARRAY OF DIETARY PREFERENCES AND COOKING METHODS. FROM THE EASE OF CROCKPOT MEALS TO THE FRESHNESS OF VEGETARIAN AND VEGAN DISHES, SMOOTHIE ENTHUSIASTS AND SNACK LOVERS WILL ALSO FIND NEW FAVORITES TO ADD TO THEIR REPERTOIRE.

CHECK OUT

THESE OTHER COOKBOOKS FROM SGT PEREZ

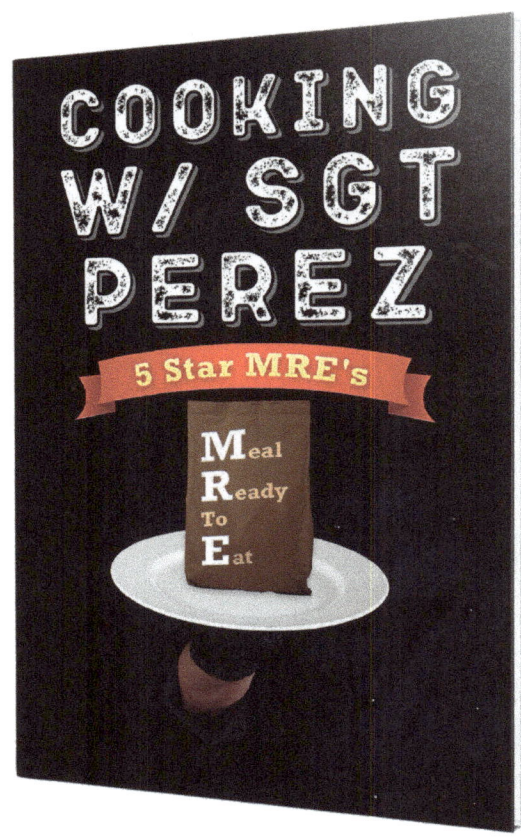

TRANSFORM THE BATTLEFIELD STAPLE INTO A GOURMET FEAST WITH "COOKING W/ SGT PEREZ 5-STAR MRES" EXPERIENCE THE RUGGED ESSENCE OF MILITARY MEALS REIMAGINED WITH A LUXURIOUS TWIST IN THIS UNIQUE COOKBOOK. EACH RECIPE ELEVATES THE SIMPLE AND QUICK MRE INTO A REFINED CULINARY DELIGHT WORTHY OF A FIVE-STAR REVIEW.

WHETHER YOU'RE A VETERAN, AN ADVENTUROUS COOK, OR SIMPLY CURIOUS ABOUT THE FUSION OF FIELD RATIONS AND FINE DINING, THIS COOKBOOK BRINGS THE THRILL OF INNOVATION TO YOUR KITCHEN. REDISCOVER FAVORITES LIKE BEEF STEW AND CHICKEN ALA KING, EACH DISH ARTFULLY ENHANCED TO ASTONISH YOUR PALATE AND IMPRESS YOUR GUESTS.

INSIDE "COOKING W/ SGT PEREZ - 5-STAR MRES," YOU'LL FIND:

CREATIVE AND UPSCALE INTERPRETATIONS OF CLASSIC MRES.
EASY-TO-FOLLOW RECIPES WITH RICH, COMPLEX FLAVORS.
TIPS FOR PLATING AND PRESENTING MEALS WITH PROFESSIONAL FLAIR.

EMBRACE THE CHALLENGE AND CHARM OF TURNING THE ORDINARY INTO THE EXTRAORDINARY. "5-STAR MRES: GOURMET EDITION" IS MORE THAN JUST A COOKBOOK— IT'S AN ADVENTURE ON YOUR DINING TABLE. GRAB YOUR COPY NOW AND ELEVATE YOUR COOKING FROM THE FIELD TO A FIVE-STAR DINING EXPERIENCE!

DO YOU LOVE

FANTASY FICTION?

CHECK OUT N. ALESSANDRO PENINTON'S NEWEST BOOK "THE ROSE IN THE GLASS DOME"

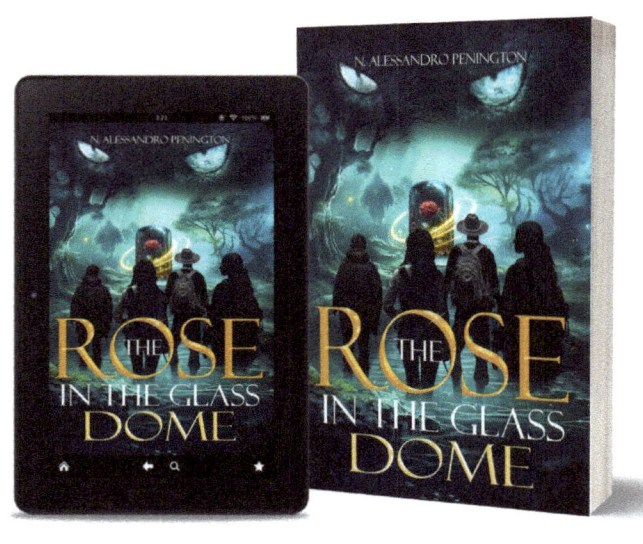

EMBARK ON A SPELLBINDING JOURNEY THROUGH THE VEILS OF DARKNESS!

PREPARE TO BE SWEPT AWAY INTO A WORLD WHERE MAGIC HOLDS SWAY AND DANGER LURKS AT EVERY SHADOWED CORNER. "THE ROSE IN THE GLASS DOME" BECKONS YOU INTO A REALM WHERE THE LINE BETWEEN REALITY AND NIGHTMARE BLURS, AND ONLY COURAGE AND CUNNING CAN CARVE A PATH TO SALVATION.

IN THE HEART OF THIS MESMERIZING TALE, A QUARTET OF INTREPID SOULS VENTURES FORTH ON A MISSION SHROUDED IN PERIL. THEIR QUEST? TO RESCUE ROSE FROM THE CLUTCHES OF A MONSTROUS TERROR. YET, FATE WEAVES A TANGLED WEB, ENSNARING THEM IN A CONSPIRACY THAT THREATENS TO PLUNGE THE ENTIRE KINGDOM INTO MADNESS.

BRIMMING WITH PULSE-POUNDING SUSPENSE AND SPINE-CHILLING TWISTS, THIS EPIC ADVENTURE IS A MASTERFUL FUSION OF ENCHANTMENT AND PERIL. FEEL THE PULSE OF EXCITEMENT QUICKEN AS YOU JOURNEY ALONGSIDE OUR HEROES, THEIR FATE INTERTWINED WITH THE DESTINY OF THE REALM ITSELF.

"THE ROSE IN THE GLASS DOME" IS A TOUR DE FORCE, BLENDING THE ALLURE OF MYSTICAL REALMS WITH THE GRITTY DETERMINATION OF THOSE WHO DARE TO DEFY DARKNESS. ARE YOU READY TO HEED THE CALL AND IMMERSE YOURSELF IN A SAGA WHERE BRAVERY KNOWS NO BOUNDS? JOIN US, AND BRACE YOURSELF FOR AN ODYSSEY THAT WILL LEAVE YOU SPELLBOUND UNTIL THE VERY LAST PAGE.

GET YOUR
COPY TODAY

ON AMAZON